Pediatric Care Guide For Emergency Medical Technicians

- ECG, Stroke, Trauma, Prehospital Infusion Reference
- Devotional for Emergency Responders

Adenosine: 0.1 mL (0.3 mg) [0.1 mg/kg: 1st dose]   0.2 mL (0.6 mg) [0.2 mg/kg: 2nd dose]
concentration: 6 mg/2 mL

Amiodarone: 0.3 mL (15 mg)
[V-Tach with Pulse: Mix 0.3 mL in 60 mL NS: 30 drops/min; 10 drop set [5 mg/kg]
concentration: 150 mg/ 3 mL

Atropine: 1 mL (0.1 mg) [0.02 mg/kg] concentration: 1 mg/10 mL maximum dose: 0.1 mg

Benadryl: Mix 50 mg/mL Benadryl + 4 mL NS: 0.3 mL (3 mg) [1 mg/kg] concentration: 50 mg/5 mL

Calcium Chloride: Mix 0.6 mL (60 mg) in 9 mL NS; Slow IV/IO [20 mg/kg]
concentration: 1000 mg/10 mL

Dextrose 10%: Mix 3 mL D50W + 12 mL NS (1.5 G) [0.5 G/kg] concentration: 1 G/2 mL

Dopamine: Mix 10 mL Dopamine + 100 mL NS: 6 drops/min. [5 mcg/kg/min]
concentration: 16,000 mcg/100 mL

Epinephrine 1:10,000: 0.3 mL (0.03 mg) [0.01 mg/kg] concentration: 1 mg/10 mL

Epinephrine 1:1000: ET: Mix 0.3 mL Epi 1:1000 + 2.7 mL NS (0.3 mg) [0.1 mg/kg]
concentration: 1 mg/mL

Epinephrine 1:1000: SQ/IM: 0.1 mL (0.1 mg)   Epi-Pen Jr. (0.15 mg)

Epinephrine: Nebulized: 2.5 mL Epi 1:1000 (2.5 mg)+ 2.5 mL NS

Fentanyl: Mix 50 mcg/mL + 4 mL NS: 0.3 mL (3 mcg) [1 mcg/kg] concentration: 50 mcg/5 mL

Fluid Bolus: 60 mL

Glucagon: 0.5 mL (0.5 mg) [0.1 mg/kg] concentration: 1 mg/mL maximum dose: 0.5 mg

Lidocaine: 0.2 mL (3 mg) [1 mg/kg] concentration: 100 mg/5 mL

Magnesium Sulfate:
concentration: 1 G/2 mL: Mix 0.3 mL (150 mg) Mag Sulfate + 60 mL NS: 60 drops/min.[10 drop set]
concentration: 2 G/50 mL: Mix 3.8 mL (150 mg) Mag Sulfate + 60 mL NS: 60 drops/min.[10 drop set]
[50 mg/kg]

Morphine: Mix 5 mg/mL Morphine in 9 mL NS: 0.6 mL (0.3 mg)   [0.1 mg/kg]
concentration: 1 mg/2mL

Narcan: 0.3 mL (0.3 mg)   [0.1 mg/kg] concentration 1 mg/mL

Newborn   3 kg

Sodium Bicarbonate: Mix 3 mL (3 mEq) Sodium Bicarbonate + 3 mL NS [1 mEq/kg]
concentration 1 mEq/mL

Solumedrol: 0.1 mL (6 mg) [2 mg/kg] concentration 62.5 mg/mL

Valium: IV/IO: 0.1 mL (0.6 mg) [0.2 mg/kg]
Rectal: 0.2 mL (1.2 mg) [0.4 mg/kg]
concentration: 5 mg/mL

Versed:
concentration: 1 mg/mL: 0.6 mL (0.6mg) [0.2 mg/kg]
concentration: 5 mg/mL: 0.1 mL (0.6 mg)   [0.2 mg/kg]

BVM: Tidal volume: 21 mL

ETT: 3.0 - 4.0   Depth: 9.5 cm

Supraglottic Airway: #1   OPA: 40 mm (Pink)   NPA:

Cardioversion: #1: 3 J #2: 6 J

 Defibrillation: #1: 6 J #2: 12 J #3: 18 J #4: 24 J #5: 30 J

Compression to Ventilation Ratio: 3:1 Compression Rate: at least 120/min;
Heart Rate< 60: Chest Compressions

" A woman giving birth to a child has pain because her time has come; but when her baby is born, she forgets the anguish because of her joy that a child is born into the world."   --- John 16:21

Adenosine: 0.1 mL (0.4 mg) [0.1 mg/kg: 1st dose]   0.3 mL (0.8 mg) [0.2 mg/kg: 2nd dose]
concentration: 6 mg/2 mL

Amiodarone: 0.4 mL (20 mg)
[V-Tach with Pulse: Mix 0.4 mL in 80 mL NS:40 drops/min;10 drop set][5 mg/kg]
concentration:150 mg/3 mL

Atropine: 1 mL (0.1 mg) [0.02 mg/kg] concentration: 1 mg/10 mL maximum dose: 0.1 mg

Benadryl: Mix 50 mg/mL Benadryl + 4 mL NS: 0.4 mL (4 mg) [1 mg/kg] concentration: 50 mg/5 mL

Calcium Chloride: Mix 0.8 mL (80 mg) in 9 mL NS; Slow IV/IO [20 mg/kg]
concentration: 1000 mg/10 mL

Dextrose 10%: Mix 4 mL D50W + 16 mL NS (2 G) [0.5 G/kg] concentration: 1 G/2 mL

Dopamine: Mix 10 mL Dopamine + 100 mL NS: 8 drops/min. [5 mcg/kg/min]
concentration: 16,000 mcg/100 mL

Epinephrine 1:10,000: 0.4 mL (0.04 mg) [0.01 mg/kg] concentration: 1 mg/10 mL

Epinephrine 1:1000: ET: Mix 0.4 mL Epi 1:1000 + 2.6 mL NS (0.4 mg) [0.1 mg/kg]
concentration: 1 mg/mL

Epinephrine 1:1000: SQ/IM: 0.1 mL (0.1 mg)   Epi-Pen Jr. (0.15 mg)

Epinephrine: Nebulized: 2.5 mL Epi 1:1000 (2.5 mg) + 2.5 mL NS

Fentanyl: Mix 50 mcg/mL + 4 mL NS: 0.4 mL (4 mcg) [1 mcg/kg] concentration: 50 mcg/5 mL

Fluid Bolus: 80 mL

Glucagon: 0.5 mL (0.5 mg) [0.1 mg/kg] concentration: 1 mg/mL maximum dose: 0.5 mg

Lidocaine: 0.2 mL (4 mg) [1 mg/kg]   concentration: 100 mg/5 mL

Magnesium Sulfate:
concentration: 1 G/2 mL: Mix 0.4 mL (200 mg) Mag Sulfate + 80 mL NS: 80 drops/min. [10 drop set]
concentration: 2 G/50 mL: Mix 5 mL (200 mg) Mag Sulfate + 80 mL NS: 80 drops/min. [10 drop set]
[50 mg/kg]

1 m/o   4 kg

Morphine: Mix 5 mg/mL Morphine in 9 mL NS: 0.8 mL (0.4 mg) [0.1 mg/kg]
concentration: 0.5 mg/mL

Narcan: 0.4 mL (0.4 mg) [0.1 mg/kg]   concentration 1 mg/mL

Sodium Bicarbonate: Mix 4 mL (4 mEq) Sodium Bicarbonate + 4 mL NS [1 mEq/kg]
concentration 1 mEq/mL

Solumedrol: 0.1 mL (8 mg) [2 mg/kg] concentration 62.5 mg/mL

Valium:
IV/IO: 0.2 mL (0.8 mg) [0.2 mg/kg]
Rectal: 0.3 mL (1.6 mg) [0.4 mg/kg]
concentration: 5 mg/mL

Versed:
concentration: 1 mg/mL: 0.8 mL (0.8mg) [0.2 mg/kg]
concentration: 5 mg/mL: 0.2 mL (0.8 mg) [0.2 mg/kg]

BVM: Tidal volume: 28 mL

ETT: 3.0 - 4.0   Depth: 10 cm

 Supraglottic Airway: #1   OPA: 40 mm (Pink)   NPA:

Cardioversion: #1: 4 J #2: 8 J

 Defibrillation: #1: 8 J #2: 16 J #3: 24 J #4: 32 J #5: 40 J

"We won't hide stories of God's blessings from our children. We will share them with the next generation." -Psalm 78:4

Adenosine: 0.2 mL (0.5 mg) [0.1 mg/kg: 1st dose]   0.3 mL (1 mg) [0.2 mg/kg: 2nd dose]
concentration: 6 mg/2 mL

Amiodarone: 0.5 mL (25 mg)
[V-Tach with Pulse: Mix 0.5 mL in 100 mL NS: 50 drops/min; 10 drop set] [5 mg/kg]
concentration: 150 mg/ 3 mL

Atropine: 1 mL (0.1 mg) [0.02 mg/kg] concentration: 1 mg/10 mL maximum dose: 0.1 mg

Benadryl: Mix 50 mg/mL Benadryl + 4 mL NS: 0.5 mL (5 mg) [1 mg/kg] concentration: 50 mg/mL

Calcium Chloride: Mix 1 mL (100 mg) in 9 mL NS; Slow IV/IO [20 mg/kg]
concentration: 1000 mg/10 mL

Dextrose 10%: Mix 5 mL D50W + 20 mL NS (2.5 G) [0.5 G/kg] concentration: 1 G/2 mL

Dopamine: Mix 10 mL Dopamine + 100 mL NS: 9 drops/min. [5 mcg/kg/min]
concentration: 16,000 mcg/100 mL

Epinephrine 1:10,000: 0.5 mL (0.05 mg) [0.01 mg/kg] concentration: 1 mg/10 mL

Epinephrine 1:1000: ET: Mix 0.5 mL Epi 1:1000 + 2.5 mL NS (0.5 mg) [0.1 mg/kg]
concentration: 1 mg/mL

Epinephrine 1:1000: SQ/IM: 0.1 mL (0.1 mg)   Epi-Pen Jr. (0.15 mg)

Epinephrine: Nebulized: 2.5 mL Epi 1:1000 (2.5 mg) + 2.5 mL NS

Fentanyl: Mix 50 mcg/mL + 4 mL NS: 0.5 mL (5 mcg) [1 mcg/kg] concentration: 50 mcg/5 mL

Fluid Bolus: 100 mL

Glucagon: 0.5 mL (0.5 mg) [0.1 mg/kg] concentration: 1 mg/mL maximum dose: 0.5 mg

Lidocaine: 0.3 mL (5 mg) [1 mg/kg] concentration: 100 mg/5 mL

Magnesium Sulfate:
concentration: 1 G/2 mL: Mix 0.5 mL (250 mg) Mag Sulfate + 100 mL NS: 100 drops/min.[10 drop set]
concentration: 2 G/50 mL: Mix 6.3 mL (250 mg) Mag Sulfate + 100 mL NS: 100 drops/min.[10 drop set]
[50 mg/kg]

Morphine: Mix 5 mg/mL Morphine in 9 mL NS: 1 mL (0.5 mg) [0.1 mg/kg]
concentration: 1 mg/2mL

Narcan: 0.5 mL (0.5 mg)   [0.1 mg/kg] concentration 1 mg/mL

2 m/o   5 kg

Sodium Bicarbonate: Mix 5 mL (5 mEq) Sodium Bicarbonate + 5 mL NS [1 mEq/kg]
concentration 1 mEq/mL

Solumedrol: 0.2 mL (10 mg) [2 mg/kg] concentration 62.5 mg/mL

Valium:
IV/IO: 0.2 mL (1 mg) [0.2 mg/kg]
Rectal: 0.4 mL (2 mg) [0.4 mg/kg]
concentration: 5 mg/mL

Versed:
concentration: 1 mg/mL: 1 mL (1 mg) [0.2 mg/kg]
concentration: 5 mg/mL: 0.2 mL (1 mg) [0.2 mg/kg]

BVM: Tidal volume: 35 mL

ETT: 4.0   Depth: 10.5 cm

Supraglottic Airway: #1.5   OPA: 40 mm (Pink)   NPA:

Cardioversion: #1: 5 J #2: 10 J

Defibrillation: #1: 10 J #2: 20 J #3: 30 J #4: 40 J #5: 50 J

" Before I formed you in the womb, I knew you." ---Jeremiah 1:5

Acetaminophen: 2.8 mL (90 mg) [15 mg/kg] concentration: 160 mg/5 mL

Adenosine: 0.2 mL (0.6 mg) [0.1 mg/kg: 1st dose]   0.4 mL (1.2 mg) [0.2 mg/kg: 2nd dose]
concentration: 6 mg/2 mL

Amiodarone: 0.6 mL (30 mg)
[V-Tach with Pulse: Mix 0.6 mL in 100 mL NS: 50 drops/min; 10 drop set][5 mg/kg]
concentration: 150 mg/ 3 mL

Atropine: 1.2 mL (.12 mg) [0.02 mg/kg] concentration: 1 mg/10 mL

Benadryl: 0.1 mL (6 mg) [1 mg/kg] concentration: 50 mg/mL

Calcium Chloride: Mix 1.2 mL (120 mg) in 8 mL NS; Slow IV/IO [20 mg/kg]
concentration: 1000 mg/10 mL

Dextrose 10%:   6 mL D50W + 24 mL NS (3 G) [0.5 G/kg] concentration: 1 G/2 mL

Dopamine: Mix 10 mL Dopamine + 100 mL NS: 11 drops/min. [5 mcg/kg/min]
concentration: 16,000 mcg/100 mL

Epinephrine 1:10,000: 0.6 mL (0.06 mg) [0.01 mg/kg]   concentration: 1 mg/10 mL

Epinephrine 1:1000: ET: Mix 0.6 mL Epi 1:1000 + 2.4 mL NS (0.6 mg) [0.1 mg/kg]
concentration: 1 mg/mL

Epinephrine 1:1000: SQ/IM: 0.1 mL (0.1 mg)   Epi-Pen Jr. (0.15 mg)

Epinephrine: Nebulized: 2.5 mL Epi 1:1000 (2.5 mg) + 2.5 mL NS

Fentanyl: 0.1 mL (6 mcg) [1 mcg/kg] concentration: 50 mcg/mL

Fluid Bolus: 120 mL

Glucagon: 0.6 mL (0.6 mg) [0.1 mg/kg] concentration: 1 mg/mL

Lidocaine: 0.3 mL (6 mg) [1 mg/kg] concentration: 100 mg/5 mL

Magnesium Sulfate:
concentration: 1 G/2 mL: Mix 0.6 mL (300 mg) Mag Sulfate + 100 mL NS: 100 drops/min.[10 drop set]
concentration: 2 G/50 mL: Mix 7.5 mL (300 mg) Mag Sulfate + 100 mL NS: 100 drops/min.[10 drop set]
[50 mg/kg]

Morphine: Mix 5 mg/mL Morphine in 9 mL NS: 1.2 mL (0.6 mg)   [0.1 mg/kg]
 concentration: 1 mg/2mL

3 m/o   6 kg

Narcan: 0.6 mL (0.6 mg) [0.1 mg/kg]   concentration 1 mg/mL

Sodium Bicarbonate: Mix 6 mL (6 mEq) Sodium Bicarbonate + 6 mL NS [1 mEq/kg]
concentration 1 mEq/mL

Solumedrol: 0.2 mL (12 mg) [2 mg/kg] concentration 62.5 mg/mL

Valium:
IV/IO: 0.2 mL (1.2 mg) [0.2 mg/kg]
Rectal: 0.5 mL (2.4 mg) [0.4 mg/kg]
concentration: 5 mg/mL

Versed:
concentration: 1 mg/mL: 1.2 mL (1.2 mg) [0.2 mg/kg]
concentration: 5 mg/mL: 0.2 mL (1.2 mg) [0.2 mg/kg]

BVM: Tidal volume: 42 mL

ETT: 4.0   Depth: 11 cm

Supraglottic Airway: #1.5   OPA: 50 mm (Blue)   NPA:

Cardioversion: #1: 6 J #2: 12 J

Defibrillation: #1: 12 J #2: 24 J #3: 36 J #4: 48 J #5: 60 J

"A father is tender and kind to his children. In the same way, the LORD is tender and kind to those who have respect for Him."   - Psalm 103:13

4 m/o   6.5 kg   (Pink)

Acetaminophen: 3 mL (97.5 mg) [15 mg/kg] concentration: 160 mg/5 mL

Adenosine: 0.2 mL (0.65 mg) [0.1 mg/kg: 1st dose]   0.4 mL (1.3 mg) [0.2 mg/kg: 2nd dose]
concentration: 6 mg/2 mL

Amiodarone: 0.7 mL (32.5 mg)
[V-Tach with Pulse: Mix 0.7 mL in 100 mL NS: 50 drops/min;10 drop set][5 mg/kg]
concentration: 150 mg/ 3 mL

Atropine: 1.3 mL (.13 mg) [0.02 mg/kg] concentration: 1 mg/10 mL

Benadryl: 0.1 mL (6.5 mg) [1 mg/kg] concentration: 50 mg/mL

Calcium Chloride: Mix 1.3 mL (130 mg) in 8 mL NS; Slow IV/IO [20 mg/kg]
concentration: 1000 mg/10 mL

Dextrose 10%: Mix 6.5 mL D50W + 26 mL NS (3.25 G) [0.5 G/kg] concentration: 1 G/2 mL

Dopamine: Mix 10 mL Dopamine + 100 mL NS: 12 drops/min. [5 mcg/kg/min]
concentration: 16,000 mcg/100 mL

Epinephrine 1:10,000: 0.7 mL (0.07 mg) [0.01 mg/kg] concentration: 1 mg/10 mL

Epinephrine 1:1000: ET: Mix 0.7 mL Epi 1:1000 + 2.3 mL NS (0.7 mg) [0.1 mg/kg]
concentration: 1 mg/mL

Epinephrine 1:1000: SQ/IM: 0.1 mL (0.1 mg)   Epi-Pen Jr. (0.15 mg)

Epinephrine: Nebulized: 2.5 mL Epi 1:1000 (2.5 mg) + 2.5 mL NS

Fentanyl: 0.1 mL (6.5 mcg) [1 mcg/kg] concentration: 50 mcg/mL

Fluid Bolus: 130 mL

Glucagon: 0.7 mL (0.7 mg) [0.1 mg/kg] concentration: 1 mg/mL

Lidocaine: 0.3 mL (6.5 mg) [1 mg/kg] concentration: 100 mg/5 mL

Magnesium Sulfate:
concentration: 1 G/2 mL: Mix 0.7 mL (325 mg) Mag Sulfate + 100 mL NS: 100 drops/min.[10 drop set]
concentration: 2 G/50 mL: Mix 8.1 mL (325 mg) Mag Sulfate + 100 mL NS: 100 drops/min.[10 drop set]
[50 mg/kg]

Morphine: Mix 5 mg/mL Morphine in 9 mL NS: 1.3 mL (0.65 mg)   [0.1 mg/kg]
concentration: 1 mg/2mL

4 m/o   6.5 kg

Narcan: 0.7 mL (0.7 mg)   [0.1 mg/kg]   concentration 1 mg/mL

Sodium Bicarbonate: Mix 6.5 mL (6.5 mEq) Sodium Bicarbonate + 6.5 mL NS [1 mEq/kg]
concentration 1 mEq/mL

Solumedrol: 0.2 mL (13 mg) [2 mg/kg] concentration 62.5 mg/mL

Valium:
IV/IO: 0.3 mL (1.3 mg) [0.2 mg/kg]
Rectal: 0.5 mL (2.6 mg)[0.4 mg/kg]
concentration: 5 mg/mL

Versed:
concentration: 1 mg/mL: 1.3 mL (1.3 mg) [0.2 mg/kg]
concentration: 5 mg/mL: 0.3 mL (1.3 mg) [0.2 mg/kg]

BVM: Tidal volume: 46 mL

ETT: 4.0   Depth: 11 cm

Supraglottic Airway: #1.5   OPA: 50 mm (Blue)   NPA: 14 F

Cardioversion: #1: 7 J #2: 13 J

Defibrillation: #1: 13 J #2: 26 J #3: 39 J #4: 52 J #5: 65 J

" Children are a gift from God. They are a reward from Him." ---Psalm 127:3

5 m/o   7 kg   (Pink)

Acetaminophen: 3.3 mL (105 mg) [15 mg/kg] concentration: 160 mg/5 mL

Adenosine: 0.2 mL (0.7 mg) [0.1 mg/kg: 1st dose]   0.5 mL (1.4 mg) [0.2 mg/kg: 2nd dose]
concentration: 6 mg/2 mL

Amiodarone: 0.7 mL (35 mg)
[V-Tach with Pulse: Mix 0.7 mL in 100 mL NS: 50 drops/min; 10 drop set][5 mg/kg]
concentration: 150 mg/ 3 mL

Atropine: 1.4 mL (.14 mg) [0.02 mg/kg] concentration: 1 mg/10 mL

Benadryl: 0.1 mL (7 mg) [1 mg/kg]   concentration: 50 mg/mL

Calcium Chloride: Mix 1.4 mL (140 mg) in 8 mL NS; Slow IV/IO [20 mg/kg]
concentration: 1000 mg/10 mL

Dextrose 10%: Mix 7 mL D50W + 28 mL NS (3.5 G) [0.5 G/kg] concentration: 1 G/2 mL

Dopamine: Mix 10 mL Dopamine + 100 mL NS: 13 drops/min. [5 mcg/kg/min]
concentration: 16,000 mcg/100 mL

Epinephrine 1:10,000: 0.7 mL (0.07 mg) [0.01 mg/kg]   concentration: 1 mg/10 mL

Epinephrine 1:1000: ET: Mix 0.7 mL Epi 1:1000 + 2.3 mL NS (0.7 mg) [0.1 mg/kg]
concentration: 1 mg/mL

Epinephrine 1:1000: SQ/IM: 0.1 mL (0.1 mg)   Epi-Pen Jr. (0.15 mg)

Epinephrine: Nebulized: 2.5 mL Epi 1:1000 (2.5 mg) + 2.5 mL NS

Fentanyl: 0.1 mL (7 mcg) [1 mcg/kg] concentration: 50 mcg/mL

Fluid Bolus: 140 mL

Glucagon: 0.7 mL (0.7 mg) [0.1 mg/kg] concentration: 1 mg/mL

Lidocaine: 0.4 mL (7 mg) [1 mg/kg] concentration: 100 mg/5 mL

Magnesium Sulfate:
concentration: 1 G/2 mL: Mix 0.7 mL (350 mg) Mag Sulfate + 100 mL NS: 100 drops/min.[10 drop set]
concentration: 2 G/50 mL: Mix 8.8 mL (350 mg) Mag Sulfate + 100 mL NS: 100 drops/min.[10 drop set]
[50 mg/kg]

Morphine: Mix 5 mg/mL Morphine in 9 mL NS: 1.4 mL (0.7 mg)   [0.1 mg/kg]
concentration: 1 mg/2mL

5 m/o   7 kg

Narcan: 0.7 mL (0.7 mg)   [0.1 mg/kg]   concentration 1 mg/mL

Sodium Bicarbonate: Mix 7 mL (7 mEq) Sodium Bicarbonate + 7 mL NS   [1 mEq/kg] concentration 1 mEq/mL

Solumedrol: 0.2 mL (14 mg) [2 mg/kg] concentration 62.5 mg/mL

Valium:
IV/IO: 0.3 mL (1.4 mg) [0.2 mg/kg]
Rectal: 0.6 mL (2.8 mg) [0.4 mg/kg]
concentration: 5 mg/mL

Versed:
concentration: 1 mg/mL: 1.4 mL (1.4 mg) [0.2 mg/kg]
concentration: 5 mg/mL: 0.3 mL (1.4 mg) [0.2 mg/kg]

BVM: Tidal volume: 49 mL

ETT: 4.0   Depth: 11.5 cm

 Supraglottic Airway: #1.5   OPA: 50 mm (Blue)   NPA: 14 F

Cardioversion: #1: 7 J #2: 14 J

 Defibrillation: #1: 14 J #2: 28 J #3: 42 J #4: 56 J #5: 70 J

" His children will be powerful in the land. Because he is honest, his children will be blessed."
Psalm 112:2

Acetaminophen: 3.5 mL (112.5 mg) [15 mg/kg] concentration: 160 mg/5 mL

Adenosine: 0.3 mL (0.75 mg) [0.1 mg/kg: 1st dose]   0.5 mL (1.5 mg) [0.2 mg/kg: 2nd dose]
concentration: 6 mg/2 mL

Amiodarone: 0.8 mL (37.5 mg)
[V-Tach with Pulse: Mix 0.8 mL in 100 mL NS: 50 drops/min;10 drop set][5 mg/kg]
concentration: 150 mg/ 3 mL

Atropine: 1.5 mL (.15 mg) [0.02 mg/kg] concentration: 1 mg/10 mL

Benadryl: 0.2 mL (7.5 mg) [1 mg/kg] concentration: 50 mg/mL

Calcium Chloride: Mix 1.5 mL (150 mg) in 8 mL NS; Slow IV/IO [20 mg/kg]
concentration: 1000 mg/10 mL

Dextrose 10%: Mix 7.5 mL D50W + 30 mL NS (3.75 G) [0.5 G/kg] concentration: 1 G/2 mL

Dopamine: Mix 10 mL Dopamine + 100 mL NS: 14 drops/min. [5 mcg/kg/min]
concentration: 16,000 mcg/100 mL

Epinephrine 1:10,000: 0.8 mL (0.075 mg) [0.01 mg/kg] concentration: 1 mg/10 mL

Epinephrine 1:1000: ET: Mix 0.8 mL Epi 1:1000 + 2.2 mL NS (0.75 mg) [0.1 mg/kg]
concentration: 1 mg/mL

Epinephrine 1:1000: SQ/IM: 0.1 mL (0.1 mg)   Epi-Pen Jr. (0.15 mg)

Epinephrine: Nebulized: 2.5 mL Epi 1:1000 (2.5 mg) + 2.5 mL NS

Fentanyl: 0.2 mL (7.5 mcg) [1 mcg/kg] concentration: 50 mcg/mL

Fluid Bolus: 150 mL

Glucagon: 0.8 mL (0.75 mg) [0.1 mg/kg] concentration: 1 mg/mL

Lidocaine: 0.4 mL (7.5 mg) [1 mg/kg] concentration: 100 mg/5 mL

Magnesium Sulfate:
concentration: 1 G/2 mL: Mix 0.8 mL (375 mg) Mag Sulfate + 100 mL NS: 100 drops/min.; 10 drop set
concentration: 2 G/50 mL: Mix 9.4 mL (375 mg) Mag Sulfate + 100 mL NS: 100 drops/min.; 10 drop set
[50 mg/kg]

6 m/o   7.5 kg

Morphine: Mix 5 mg/mL Morphine in 9 mL NS: 1.5 mL (0.75 mg)   [0.1 mg/kg]
concentration: 1 mg/2mL

Narcan: 0.8 mL (0.75 mg)   [0.1 mg/kg]   concentration 1 mg/mL

Sodium Bicarbonate: Mix 7.5 mL (7.5 mEq) Sodium Bicarbonate + 7.5 mL NS   [1 mEq/kg]
concentration 1 mEq/mL

Solumedrol: 0.2 mL (15 mg) [2 mg/kg] concentration 62.5 mg/mL

Valium:
IV/IO: 0.3 mL (1.5 mg) [0.2 mg/kg]
Rectal: 0.6 mL (3 mg) [0.4 mg/kg]
concentration: 5 mg/mL

Versed:
concentration: 1 mg/mL: 1.5 mL (1.5 mg) [0.2 mg/kg]
concentration: 5 mg/mL: 0.3 mL (1.5 mg) [0.2 mg/kg]

BVM: Tidal volume: 52.5 mL

ETT: 4.0   Depth: 11.5- 12 cm

 Supraglottic Airway: #1.5   OPA: 50 mm (Blue)   NPA: 14 F

Cardioversion: #1: 8 J #2: 15 J

 Defibrillation: #1: 15 J #2: 30 J #3: 45 J #4: 60 J #5: 75 J

" What then is this child going to be? For the LORD's hand was with him." ---Luke 1:66

Acetaminophen: 3.8 mL (120mg) [15 mg/kg] concentration: 160 mg/5 mL

Adenosine: 0.3 mL (0.8 mg) [0.1 mg/kg: 1st dose]   0.5 mL (1.6 mg) [0.2 mg/kg: 2nd dose] concentration: 6 mg/2 mL

Amiodarone: 0.8 mL (40 mg)
[V-Tach with Pulse: Mix 0.8 mL in 100 mL NS: 50 drops/min; 10 drop set]   [5 mg/kg] concentration: 150 mg/ 3 mL

Atropine: 1.6 mL (.16 mg) [0.02 mg/kg] concentration: 1 mg/10 mL

Benadryl: 0.2 mL (8 mg) [1 mg/kg]   concentration: 50 mg/mL

Calcium Chloride: Mix 1.6 mL (160 mg) in 8 mL NS; Slow IV/IO [20 mg/kg] concentration: 1000 mg/10 mL

Dextrose 10%: Mix 8 mL D50W + 32 mL NS (4 G) [0.5 G/kg] concentration: 1 G/2 mL

Dopamine: Mix 10 mL Dopamine + 100 mL NS: 15 drops/min. [5 mcg/kg/min] concentration: 16,000 mcg/100 mL

Epinephrine 1:10,000: 0.8 mL (0.08 mg) [0.01 mg/kg]   concentration: 1 mg/10 mL

Epinephrine 1:1000: ET: Mix 0.8 mL Epi 1:1000 + 2.2 mL NS (0.8 mg) [0.1 mg/kg] concentration: 1 mg/mL

Epinephrine 1:1000: SQ/IM: 0.1 mL (0.1 mg)   Epi-Pen Jr. (0.15 mg)

Epinephrine: Nebulized: 2.5 mL Epi 1:1000 (2.5 mg) + 2.5 mL NS

Fentanyl: 0.2 mL (8 mcg) [1 mcg/kg] concentration: 50 mcg/mL

Fluid Bolus: 160 mL

Glucagon: 0.8 mL (0.8 mg) [0.1 mg/kg] concentration: 1 mg/mL

Ibuprofen: 4 mL (80 mg) [10 mg/kg] concentration: 20 mg/mL

Lidocaine: 0.4 mL (8 mg) [1 mg/kg] concentration: 100 mg/5 mL

Magnesium Sulfate:
concentration: 1 G/2 mL: Mix 0.8 mL (400 mg) Mag Sulfate + 100 mL NS: 100 drops/min.; 10 drop set
concentration: 2 G/50 mL: Mix 10 mL (400 mg) Mag Sulfate + 100 mL NS: 100 drops/min.; 10 drop set
[50 mg/kg]

7 m/o   8 kg

Morphine: Mix 5 mg/mL Morphine in 9 mL NS: 1.6 mL (0.8 mg)   [0.1 mg/kg]
concentration: 1 mg/2mL

Narcan: 0.8 mL (0.8 mg)   [0.1 mg/kg]   concentration 1 mg/mL

Sodium Bicarbonate: Mix 8 mL (8 mEq) Sodium Bicarbonate + 8 mL NS   [1 mEq/kg]
concentration 1 mEq/mL

Solumedrol: 0.3 mL (16 mg) [2 mg/kg]   concentration 62.5 mg/mL

Valium:
IV/IO: 0.3 mL (1.6 mg) [0.2 mg/kg]
Rectal: 0.6 mL (3.2 mg) [0.4 mg/kg]
concentration: 5 mg/mL

Versed:
concentration: 1 mg/mL: 1.6 mL (1.6 mg) [0.2 mg/kg]
concentration: 5 mg/mL: 0.3 mL (1.6 mg) [0.2 mg/kg]

Zofran: Mix 0.4 mL (0.8 mg) Zofran + 2 mL NS Slow IVP [0.1 mg/kg] concentration: 2 mg/mL

BVM: Tidal volume: 56 mL

ETT: 4.0   Depth: 12 cm

 Supraglottic Airway: #1.5   OPA: 50 mm (Blue)   NPA: 16 F

Cardioversion: #1: 8 J #2: 16 J

 Defibrillation: #1: 16 J #2: 32 J #3: 48 J #4: 64 J #5: 80 J

"Jesus took the little girl by the hand and healed her." -Mark 5:41

8 m/o   8.5 kg   (Red)

Acetaminophen: 4 mL (127.5 mg) [15 mg/kg] concentration: 160 mg/5 mL

Adenosine: 0.3 mL (0.85 mg) [0.1 mg/kg: 1st dose]   0.6 mL (1.7 mg) [0.2 mg/kg: 2nd dose]
concentration: 6 mg/2 mL

Amiodarone: 0.9 mL (42.5 mg)
[V-Tach with Pulse: Mix 0.9 mL in 100 mL NS: 50 drops/min;10 drop set] [5 mg/kg]
concentration:150 mg/ 3 mL

Atropine: 1.7 mL (.17 mg) [0.02 mg/kg] concentration: 1 mg/10 mL

Benadryl: 0.2 mL (8.5 mg) [1 mg/kg]   concentration: 50 mg/mL

Calcium Chloride: Mix 1.7 mL (170 mg) in 8 mL NS; Slow IV/IO [20 mg/kg]
concentration: 1000 mg/10 mL

Dextrose 10%: Mix 8.5 mL D50W + 34 mL NS (4.25 G) [0.5 G/kg] concentration: 1 G/2 mL

Dopamine: Mix 10 mL Dopamine + 100 mL NS: 16 drops/min. [5 mcg/kg/min]
concentration: 16,000 mcg/100 mL

Epinephrine 1:10,000: 0.9 mL (0.085 mg) [0.01 mg/kg]   concentration: 1 mg/10 mL

Epinephrine 1:1000: ET: Mix 0.9 mL Epi 1:1000 + 2.1 mL NS (0.85 mg) [0.1 mg/kg]
concentration: 1 mg/mL

Epinephrine 1:1000: SQ/IM: 0.1 mL (0.1 mg)   Epi-Pen Jr. (0.15 mg)

Epinephrine: Nebulized: 2.5 mL Epi 1:1000 (2.5 mg) + 2.5 mL NS

Fentanyl: 0.2 mL (8.5 mcg) [1 mcg/kg] concentration: 50 mcg/mL

Fluid Bolus: 170 mL

Glucagon: 0.9 mL (0.85 mg) [0.1 mg/kg] concentration: 1 mg/mL

Ibuprofen: 4.3 mL (85 mg) [10 mg/kg]   concentration: 20 mg/mL

Lidocaine: 0.4 mL (8.5 mg) [1 mg/kg]   concentration: 100 mg/5 mL

Magnesium Sulfate:
concentration: 1 G/2 mL: Mix 0.9 mL (425 mg) Mag Sulfate + 100 mL NS: 100 drops/min.; 10 drop set
concentration: 2 G/50 mL: Mix 10.6 mL (425 mg) Mag Sulfate + 100 mL NS: 100 drops/min.;10 drop set
[50 mg/kg]

8 m/o   8.5 kg

Morphine: Mix 5 mg/mL Morphine in 9 mL NS: 1.7 mL (0.85 mg)   [0.1 mg/kg]
concentration: 1 mg/2mL

Narcan: 0.9 mL (0.85 mg)   [0.1 mg/kg]   concentration 1 mg/mL

Sodium Bicarbonate: Mix 8.5 mL (8.5 mEq) Sodium Bicarbonate + 8.5 mL NS [1 mEq/kg]
concentration 1 mEq/mL

Solumedrol: 0.3 mL (17 mg) [2 mg/kg]   concentration 62.5 mg/mL

Valium:
IV/IO: 0.3 mL (1.7 mg) [0.2 mg/kg]
Rectal: 0.7 mL (3.4 mg) [0.4 mg/kg]
concentration: 5 mg/mL

Versed:
concentration: 1 mg/mL: 1.7 mL (1.7 mg) [0.2 mg/kg]
concentration: 5 mg/mL: 0.3 mL (1.7 mg) [0.2 mg/kg]

Zofran: Mix 0.4 mL (0.85 mg) Zofran + 2 mL NS Slow IVP [0.1 mg/kg] concentration: 2 mg/mL

BVM: Tidal volume: 59.5 mL

ETT: 4.0   Depth: 12 cm

Supraglottic Airway: #1.5   OPA: 50 mm (Blue)   NPA: 16 F

Cardioversion: #1: 9 J #2: 17 J

Defibrillation: #1: 17 J #2: 34 J #3: 51 J #4: 68 J #5: 85 J

" Jesus said, 'Let the little children come to Me, and do not hinder them, for the kingdom of God belongs to them.'"   Mark 10:14

Acetaminophen: 4.2 mL (135 mg) [15 mg/kg]   concentration: 160 mg/5 mL

Adenosine: 0.3 mL (0.9 mg) [0.1 mg/kg: 1st dose]   0.6 mL (1.8 mg) [0.2 mg/kg: 2nd dose]
concentration: 6 mg/2 mL

Amiodarone: 0.9 mL (45 mg)
[V-Tach with Pulse: Mix 0.9 mL in 100 mL NS; 50 drops/min; 10 drop set] [5 mg/kg]
concentration: 150 mg/ 3 mL

Atropine: 1.8 mL (0.18 mg) [0.02 mg/kg] concentration: 1 mg/10 mL

Benadryl: 0.2 mL (9 mg) [1 mg/kg] concentration: 50 mg/mL

Calcium Chloride: Mix 1.8 mL (180 mg) in 8 mL NS; Slow IV/IO [20 mg/kg]
concentration: 1000 mg/10 mL

Dextrose 10%: Mix 9 mL D50W + 36 mL NS (4.5 G) [0.5 G/kg] concentration: 1 G/2 mL

Dopamine: Mix 10 mL Dopamine + 100 mL NS: 17 drops/min. [5 mcg/kg/min]
concentration: 16,000 mcg/100 mL

Epinephrine 1:10,000: 0.9 mL (0.09 mg) [0.01 mg/kg]   concentration: 1 mg/10 mL

Epinephrine 1:1000: ET: Mix 0.9 mL Epi 1:1000 + 2.1 mL NS (0.9 mg) [0.1 mg/kg]
concentration: 1 mg/mL

Epinephrine 1:1000: SQ/IM: 0.1 mL (0.1 mg)   Epi-Pen Jr. (0.15 mg)

Epinephrine: Nebulized: 2.5 mL Epi 1:1000 (2.5 mg) + 2.5 mL NS

Fentanyl: 0.2 mL (9 mcg) [1 mcg/kg] concentration: 50 mcg/mL

Fluid Bolus: 180 mL

Glucagon: 0.9 mL (0.9 mg) [0.1 mg/kg] concentration: 1 mg/mL

Ibuprofen: 4.5 mL (90 mg) [10 mg/kg] concentration: 20 mg/mL

Lidocaine: 0.5 mL (9 mg) [1 mg/kg] concentration: 100 mg/5 mL

Magnesium Sulfate
concentration: 1 G/2 mL: Mix 0.9 mL (450 mg) Mag Sulfate + 100 mL NS: 100 drops/min.; 10 drop set
concentration: 2 G/50 mL: Mix 11.3 mL (450 mg) Mag Sulfate + 100 mL NS: 100 drops/min.;10 drop set
[50 mg/kg]

9 m/o   9 kg

Morphine: Mix 5 mg/mL Morphine in 9 mL NS: 1.8 mL (0.9 mg)   [0.1 mg/kg]
concentration: 1 mg/2mL

Narcan: 0.9 mL (0.9 mg)   [0.1 mg/kg] concentration 1 mg/mL

Sodium Bicarbonate: Mix 9 mL (9 mEq) Sodium Bicarbonate + 9 mL NS   [1 mEq/kg]
concentration 1 mEq/mL

Solumedrol: 0.3 mL (18 mg) [2 mg/kg] concentration 62.5 mg/mL

Valium:
IV/IO: 0.4 mL (1.8 mg) [0.2 mg/kg]
Rectal: 0.7 mL (3.6 mg) [0.4 mg/kg]
concentration: 5 mg/mL

Versed:
concentration: 1 mg/mL: 1.8 mL (1.8 mg) [0.2 mg/kg]
concentration: 5 mg/mL: 0.4 mL (1.8 mg) [0.2 mg/kg]

Zofran: Mix 0.5 mL (0.9 mg) Zofran + 2 mL NS Slow IVP   [0.1 mg/kg]   concentration: 2 mg/mL

BVM: Tidal volume: 63 mL

ETT: 4.0   Depth: 12.5 cm

Supraglottic Airway: #1.5   OPA: 50 mm (Blue)   NPA: 16 F

Cardioversion: #1: 9 J #2: 18 J

Defibrillation: #1: 18 J #2: 36 J #3: 54 J #4: 72 J #5: 90 J

" You know how to give good gifts to your children. How much more will your Father in heaven give the Holy Spirit to those who ask Him!"   -Luke 11:13

Acetaminophen: 4.5 mL (142.5 mg) [15 mg/kg] concentration: 160 mg/5 mL

Adenosine: 0.3 mL (0.95 mg) [0.1 mg/kg: 1st dose]   0.6 mL (1.9 mg) [0.2 mg/kg: 2nd dose] concentration: 6 mg/2 mL

Amiodarone: 1 mL (47.5 mg)
[V-Tach with Pulse: Mix 1 mL in 100 mL NS: 50 drops/min; 10 drop set]   [5 mg/kg]
concentration: 150 mg/ 3 mL

Atropine: 1.9 mL (.19 mg) [0.02 mg/kg] concentration: 1 mg/10 mL

Benadryl: 0.2 mL (9.5 mg) [1 mg/kg] concentration: 50 mg/mL

Calcium Chloride: Mix 1.9 mL (190 mg) in 8 mL NS; Slow IV/IO [20 mg/kg]
concentration: 1000 mg/10 mL

Dextrose 10%: Mix 9.5 mL D50W + 38 mL NS (4.75 G) [0.5 G/kg] concentration: 1 G/2 mL

Dopamine: Mix 10 mL Dopamine + 100 mL NS: 18 drops/min. [5 mcg/kg/min]
concentration: 16,000 mcg/100 mL

Epinephrine 1:10,000: 1 mL (0.095 mg) [0.01 mg/kg] concentration: 1 mg/10 mL

Epinephrine 1:1000: ET: Mix 1 mL Epi 1:1000 + 2 mL NS (0.95 mg) [0.1 mg/kg] concentration: 1 mg/mL

Epinephrine 1:1000: SQ/IM: 0.1 mL (0.1 mg)   Epi-Pen Jr. (0.15 mg)

Epinephrine: Nebulized: 2.5 mL Epi 1:1000 (2.5 mg) + 2.5 mL NS

Fentanyl: 0.2 mL (9.5 mcg) [1 mcg/kg] concentration: 50 mcg/mL

Fluid Bolus: 190 mL

Glucagon: 1 mL (0.95 mg) [0.1 mg/kg] concentration: 1 mg/mL

Ibuprofen: 4.8 mL (95 mg) [10 mg/kg] concentration: 20 mg/mL

Lidocaine: 0.5 mL (9.5 mg) [1 mg/kg] concentration: 100 mg/5 mL

Magnesium Sulfate:
concentration: 1 G/2 mL: Mix 1 mL (475 mg) Mag Sulfate + 100 mL NS: 100 drops/min.; 10 drop set
concentration: 2 G/50 mL: Mix 11.9 mL (475 mg) Mag Sulfate + 100 mL NS: 100 drops/min.;10 drop set
[50 mg/kg]

Morphine: Mix 5 mg/mL Morphine in 9 mL NS: 1.9 mL (0.95 mg)   [0.1 mg/kg]
concentration: 1 mg/2mL

10 m/o   9.5 kg

Narcan: 1 mL (0.95 mg)   [0.1 mg/kg]   concentration 1 mg/mL

Sodium Bicarbonate: Mix 9.5 mL (9.5 mEq) Sodium Bicarbonate + 9.5 mL NS   [1 mEq/kg] concentration 1 mEq/mL

Solumedrol: 0.3 mL (19 mg) [2 mg/kg] concentration 62.5 mg/mL

Valium:
IV/IO: 0.4 mL (1.9 mg) [0.2 mg/kg]
Rectal: 0.8 mL (3.8 mg) [0.4 mg/kg]
concentration: 5 mg/mL

Versed:
concentration: 1 mg/mL: 1.9 mL (1.9 mg) [0.2 mg/kg]
concentration: 5 mg/mL: 0.4 mL (1.9 mg) [0.2 mg/kg]

Zofran: Mix 0.5 mL (0.95 mg) Zofran + 2 mL NS Slow IVP [0.1 mg/kg] concentration: 2 mg/mL

BVM: Tidal volume: 66.5 mL

ETT: 4.0 - 4.5   Depth: 13 cm

Supraglottic Airway: #1.5   OPA: 50 mm (Blue)   NPA: 16 F

Cardioversion: #1: 10 J #2: 19 J

Defibrillation: #1: 19 J #2: 38 J #3: 57 J #4: 76 J #5: 95 J

" Your Father in Heaven is not willing that any of these little ones be lost." ---Matthew 18:14

11 m/o   10 kg   (Purple)

Acetaminophen: 4.7 mL (150 mg) [15 mg/kg] concentration: 160 mg/5 mL

Adenosine: 0.3 mL (1 mg) [0.1 mg/kg: 1st dose]   0.7 mL (2 mg) [0.2 mg/kg:2nd dose]
concentration: 6 mg/2 mL

Amiodarone: 1 mL (50 mg)
[V-Tach with Pulse: Mix 1 mL in 100 mL NS: 50 drops/min; 10 drop set]   [5 mg/kg]
concentration: 150 mg/ 3 mL

Atropine: 2 mL (0.2 mg) [0.02 mg/kg] concentration: 1 mg/10 mL

Benadryl: 0.2 mL (10 mg) [1 mg/kg] concentration: 50 mg/mL

Calcium Chloride: Mix 2 mL (200 mg) in 8 mL NS; Slow IV/IO [20 mg/kg]
concentration: 1000 mg/10 mL

Dextrose 10%: Mix 10 mL D50W + 40 mL NS (5 G) [0.5 G/kg] concentration: 1 G/2 mL

Dopamine: Mix 10 mL Dopamine + 100 mL NS: 19 drops/min. [5 mcg/kg/min]
concentration: 16,000 mcg/100 mL

Epinephrine 1:10,000: 1 mL (0.1 mg) [0.01 mg/kg] concentration: 1 mg/10 mL

Epinephrine 1:1000: ET: Mix 1 mL Epi 1:1000 + 2 mL NS (1 mg) [0.1 mg/kg] concentration: 1 mg/mL

Epinephrine 1:1000: SQ/IM: 0.1 mL (0.1 mg)   Epi-Pen Jr. (0.15 mg)

Epinephrine: Nebulized: 2.5 mL Epi 1:1000 (2.5 mg) + 2.5 mL NS

Fentanyl: 0.2 mL (10 mcg) [1 mcg/kg] concentration: 50 mcg/mL

Fluid Bolus: 200 mL

Glucagon: 1 mL (1 mg) [0.1 mg/kg] concentration: 1 mg/mL

Ibuprofen: 5 mL (100 mg) [10 mg/kg] concentration: 20 mg/mL

Lidocaine: 0.5 mL (10 mg) [1 mg/kg] concentration: 100 mg/5 mL

Magnesium Sulfate:
concentration: 1 G/2 mL: Mix 1 mL (500 mg) Mag Sulfate + 100 mL NS: 100 drops/min.; 10 drop set
concentration: 2 G/50 mL: Mix 12.5 mL (500 mg) Mag Sulfate + 100 mL NS: 100 drops/min.;10 drop set
[50 mg/kg]

Morphine: Mix 5 mg/mL Morphine in 9 mL NS: 2 mL (1 mg)   [0.1 mg/kg]
concentration: 1 mg/2mL

11 m/o   10 kg

Narcan: 1 mL (1 mg)   [0.1 mg/kg]   concentration 1 mg/mL

Sodium Bicarbonate: Mix 10 mL (10 mEq) Sodium Bicarbonate + 10 mL NS   [1 mEq/kg] concentration 1 mEq/mL

Solumedrol: 0.3 mL (20 mg) [2 mg/kg] concentration 62.5 mg/mL

Valium:
IV/IO: 0.4 mL (2 mg) [0.2 mg/kg]
Rectal: 0.8 mL (4 mg) [0.4 mg/kg]
concentration: 5 mg/mL

Versed:
concentration: 1 mg/mL: 2 mL (2 mg) [0.2 mg/kg]
concentration: 5 mg/mL: 0.4 mL (2 mg) [0.2 mg/kg]

Zofran: Mix 0.5 mL (1 mg) Zofran + 2 mL NS: Slow IVP [0.1 mg/kg]   concentration: 2 mg/mL

BVM: Tidal volume: 70 mL

ETT: 4.0 – 4.5   Depth: 13 cm

Supraglottic Airway: #1.5   OPA: 60 mm (Black)   NPA: 18 F

Cardioversion: #1: 10 J #2: 20 J

Defibrillation: #1: 20 J #2: 40 J #3: 60 J #4: 80 J #5: 100 J

"Be strong and courageous. The LORD your GOD will go with you. He will never leave you or desert you."   -Deuteronomy 31:6

Acetaminophen: 5.2 mL (165 mg) [15 mg/kg] concentration: 160 mg/5 mL

Adenosine: 0.4 mL (1.1 mg) [0.1 mg/kg: 1st dose]   0.7 mL (2.2 mg) [0.2 mg/kg: 2nd dose] concentration: 6 mg/2 mL

Amiodarone:1.1 mL(55 mg)
[V-Tach with Pulse: Mix 1.1 mL in 100mL NS;50 drops/min;10 drop set]   [5 mg/kg] concentration:150 mg/3 mL

Atropine: 2.2 mL (0.22 mg) [0.02 mg/kg] concentration: 1 mg/10 mL

Benadryl: 0.2 mL (11 mg) [1 mg/kg]   concentration: 50 mg/mL

Calcium Chloride: Mix 2.2 mL (220 mg) in 7 mL NS; Slow IV/IO [20 mg/kg] concentration: 1000 mg/10 mL

Dextrose 25%: Mix 11 mL D50W + 11 mL NS (5.5 G) [0.5 G/kg]   concentration: 1 G/2 mL

Dopamine: Mix 10 mL Dopamine + 100 mL NS: 21 drops/min. [5 mcg/kg/min] concentration: 16,000 mcg/100 mL

Epinephrine 1:10,000: 1.1 mL (0.11 mg) [0.01 mg/kg] concentration: 1 mg/10 mL

Epinephrine 1:1000: ET: Mix 1.1 mL Epi 1:1000 + 1.9 mL NS (1 mg) [0.1 mg/kg] concentration: 1 mg/mL

Epinephrine 1:1000: SQ/IM: 0.1 mL (0.1 mg)   Epi-Pen Jr. (0.15 mg)

Epinephrine: Nebulized: 2.5 mL Epi 1:1000 (2.5 mg) + 2.5 mL NS

Fentanyl: 0.2 mL (11 mcg) [1 mcg/kg] concentration: 50 mcg/mL

Fluid Bolus: 220 mL

Glucagon: 1 mL (1 mg) [0.1 mg/kg] concentration: 1 mg/mL

Ibuprofen: 5.5 mL (110 mg) [10 mg/kg] concentration: 20 mg/mL

Lidocaine: 0.6 mL (11 mg) [1 mg/kg] concentration: 100 mg/5 mL

Magnesium Sulfate:
concentration: 1 G/2 mL: Mix 1.1 mL (550 mg) Mag Sulfate + 100 mL NS: 100 drops/min.; 10 drop set
concentration: 2 G/50 mL: Mix 13.8 mL (550 mg) Mag Sulfate + 100 mL NS: 100 drops/min.;10 drop set
[50 mg/kg]

1 y/o   11 kg

Morphine: Mix 5 mg/mL Morphine in 9 mL NS: 2.2 mL (1.1 mg)   [0.1 mg/kg]
concentration: 1 mg/2mL

Narcan: 1.1 mL (1.1 mg)   [0.1 mg/kg]   concentration 1 mg/mL

Sodium Bicarbonate: Mix 11 mL (11 mEq) Sodium Bicarbonate + 11 mL NS   [1 mEq/kg]
concentration 1 mEq/mL

Solumedrol: 0.4 mL (22 mg)   [2 mg/kg]   concentration 62.5 mg/mL

Valium:
IV/IO: 0.4 mL (2.2 mg) [0.2 mg/kg]
Rectal: 0.9 mL (4.4 mg) [0.4 mg/kg]
concentration: 5 mg/mL

Versed:
concentration: 1 mg/mL: 2.2 mL (2.2 mg) [0.2 mg/kg]
concentration: 5 mg/mL: 0.4 mL (2.2 mg) [0.2 mg/kg]

Zofran: Mix 0.6 mL (1.1 mg) Zofran in 2 mL NS Slow IVP [0.1 mg/kg]   concentration: 2 mg/mL

BVM: Tidal volume: 77 mL

 ETT: 4.0- 4.5   Depth: 13.5 cm

Supraglottic Airway: #2   OPA: 60 mm (Black)   NPA: 18 F

Cardioversion: #1: 11 J #2: 22 J

 Defibrillation: #1: 22 J #2: 44 J #3: 66 J #4: 88 J #5: 110 J

" Jesus took the children in His arms, put His hands on them, and blessed them." ---Mark 10:16

2 y/o   13 kg   (Yellow)

Acetaminophen: 6.1 mL (195 mg) [15 mg/kg] concentration: 160 mg/5 mL

Adenosine: 0.4 mL (1.3 mg) [0.1 mg/kg: 1st dose]   0.9 mL (2.6 mg) [0.2 mg/kg: 2nd dose] concentration: 6 mg/2 mL

Amiodarone: 1.3 mL (65 mg)
[V-Tach with Pulse: Mix 1.3 mL in 100 mL NS: 50 drops/min; 10 drop set]   [5 mg/kg] concentration: 150 mg/ 3 mL

Atropine: 2.6 mL (0.26 mg) [0.02 mg/kg] concentration: 1 mg/10 mL

Benadryl: 0.3 mL (13 mg) [1 mg/kg] concentration: 50 mg/mL

Calcium Chloride: Mix 2.6 mL (260 mg) in 7 mL NS; Slow IV/IO [20 mg/kg] concentration: 1000 mg/10 mL

Dextrose 25%: Mix 13 mL D50W + 13 mL NS (6.5 G) [0.5 G/kg] concentration: 1 G/2 mL

Dopamine: Mix 10 mL Dopamine + 100 mL NS: 24 drops/min. [5 mcg/kg/min] concentration: 16,000 mcg/100 mL

Epinephrine 1:10,000: 1.3 mL (0.13 mg) [0.01 mg/kg]   concentration: 1 mg/10 mL

Epinephrine 1:1000: ET: Mix 1.3 mL Epi 1:1000 + 1.7 mL NS (1.3 mg)   [0.1 mg/kg] concentration: 1 mg/mL

Epinephrine 1:1000: SQ/IM: 0.2 mL (0.2 mg)   Epi-Pen Jr. (0.15 mg)

Epinephrine: Nebulized: 2.5 mL Epi 1:1000 (2.5 mg) + 2.5 mL NS

Fentanyl: 0.3 mL (13 mcg) [1 mcg/kg] concentration: 50 mcg/mL

Fluid Bolus: 260 mL

Glucagon: 1 mL (1 mg)   [0.1 mg/kg] concentration: 1 mg/mL

Ibuprofen: 6.5 mL (130 mg) [10 mg/kg] concentration: 20 mg/mL

Lidocaine: 0.7 mL (13 mg) [1 mg/kg] concentration: 100 mg/5 mL

Magnesium Sulfate:
concentration: 1 G/2 mL: Mix 1.3 mL (650 mg) Mag Sulfate + 100 mL NS: 100 drops/min.; 10 drop set
concentration: 2 G/50 mL: Mix 16.3 mL (650 mg) Mag Sulfate + 100 mL NS: 100 drops/min.;10 drop set
[50 mg/kg]

2 y/o   13 kg

Morphine: Mix 5 mg/mL Morphine in 9 mL NS: 2.6 mL (1.3 mg)   [0.1 mg/kg]
concentration: 1 mg/2mL

Narcan: 1.3 mL (1.3 mg)   [0.1 mg/kg]   concentration 1 mg/mL

Sodium Bicarbonate: Mix 13 mL (13 mEq) Sodium Bicarbonate + 13 mL NS   [1 mEq/kg]
concentration 1 mEq/mL

Solumedrol: 0.4 mL (26 mg) [2 mg/kg] concentration 62.5 mg/mL

Valium:
IV/IO: 0.5 mL (2.6 mg) [0.2 mg/kg]
Rectal: 1 mL (5.2 mg) [0.4 mg/kg]
concentration: 5 mg/mL

Versed:
concentration: 1 mg/mL: 2.6 mL (2.6 mg) [0.2 mg/kg]
concentration: 5 mg/mL: 0.5 mL (2.6 mg) [0.2 mg/kg]

Zofran: Mix 0.7 mL (1.3 mg) in 2 mL NS, Slow IVP   [0.1 mg/kg]   concentration: 2 mg/mL

BVM: Tidal volume: 91 mL

ETT: 5.0   Depth: 14 cm

Supraglottic Airway: #2   OPA: 60 mm (Black)   NPA: 20 F

Cardioversion: #1: 13 J #2: 26 J

Defibrillation: #1: 26 J #2: 52 J #3: 78 J #4: 104 J #5: 130 J

"God has appointed people who have the gift of healing and are able to help others."
1 Corinthians 12:28

Acetaminophen: 7.5 mL (240 mg) [15 mg/kg] concentration: 160 mg/5 mL

Adenosine: 0.5 mL (1.6 mg) [0.1 mg/kg: 1st dose]   1.1 mL (3.2 mg) [0.2 mg/kg: 2nd dose]
concentration: 6 mg/2 mL

Amiodarone: 1.6 mL (80 mg)
[V-Tach with Pulse: Mix 1.6 mL in 100 mL NS: 50 drops/min; 10 drop set]   [5 mg/kg]
concentration: 150 mg/ 3 mL

Atropine: 3.2 mL (0.32 mg) [0.02 mg/kg] concentration: 1 mg/10 mL

Benadryl: 0.3 mL (16 mg) [1 mg/kg] concentration: 50 mg/mL

Calcium Chloride: Mix 3.2 mL (320 mg) in 6 mL NS; Slow IV/IO [20 mg/kg]
concentration: 1000 mg/10 mL

Dextrose 25%: Mix 16 mL D50W + 16 mL NS (8 G) [0.5 G/kg] concentration: 1 G/2 mL

Dopamine: Mix 10 mL Dopamine + 100 mL NS: 30 drops/min. [5 mcg/kg/min]
concentration: 16,000 mcg/100 mL

Epinephrine 1:10,000: 1.6 mL (0.16 mg) [0.01 mg/kg]   concentration: 1 mg/10 mL

Epinephrine 1:1000: ET: Mix 1.6 mL Epi 1:1000 + 1.4 mL NS (1.6 mg) [0.1 mg/kg]
concentration: 1 mg/mL

Epinephrine 1:1000: SQ/IM: 0.2 mL (0.2 mg)   Epi-Pen Jr. (0.15 mg)

Epinephrine: Nebulized: 5 mL Epi 1:1000 (0.5 mg)

Fentanyl: 0.3 mL (16 mcg) [1 mcg/kg] concentration: 50 mcg/mL

Fluid Bolus: 320 mL

Glucagon: 1 mL (1 mg) [0.1 mg/kg] concentration: 1 mg/mL

Ibuprofen: 8 mL (160 mg) [10 mg/kg] concentration: 20 mg/mL

Lidocaine: 0.8 mL (16 mg) [1 mg/kg] concentration: 100 mg/5 mL

Magnesium Sulfate:
concentration: 1 G/2 mL: Mix 1.6 mL (800 mg) Mag Sulfate + 100 mL NS: 100 drops/min.; 10 drop set
concentration: 2 G/50 mL: Mix 20 mL (800 mg) Mag Sulfate + 100 mL NS: 100 drops/min.; 10 drop set
[50 mg/kg]

3 y/o   16 kg

Morphine: Mix 5 mg/mL Morphine in 9 mL NS: 3.2 mL (1.6 mg)   [0.1 mg/kg]
concentration: 1 mg/2mL

Narcan: 1.6 mL (1.6 mg)   [0.1 mg/kg]   concentration 1 mg/mL

Sodium Bicarbonate: 16 mL (16 mEq)   [1 mEq/kg]   concentration 1 mEq/mL

Solumedrol: 0.5 mL (32 mg) [2 mg/kg] concentration 62.5 mg/mL

Valium:
IV/IO: 0.6 mL (3.2 mg) [0.2 mg/kg]
Rectal: 1.3 mL (6.4 mg) [0.4 mg/kg]
concentration: 5 mg/mL

Versed:
concentration: 1 mg/mL: 3.2 mL (3.2 mg) [0.2 mg/kg]
concentration: 5 mg/mL: 0.6 mL (3.2 mg) [0.2 mg/kg]

Zofran: Mix 0.8 mL (1.6 mg) in 2 mL NS, Slow IVP   [0.1 mg/kg]   concentration: 2 mg/mL

BVM: Tidal volume: 112 mL

ETT: 5.0   Depth: 14.5 cm

Supraglottic Airway: #2   OPA: 60 mm (Black)   NPA: 22 F

Cardioversion: #1: 16 J #2: 32 J

Defibrillation: #1: 32 J #2: 64 J #3: 96 J #4: 128 J #5: 160 J

" Jesus said, 'Whoever welcomes one of these little children in My Name, welcomes Me.'"
Mark 9:37

4 y/o   19 kg   (Blue)

Acetaminophen: 8.9 mL (285 mg) [15 mg/kg]   concentration: 160 mg/5 mL

Adenosine: 0.6 mL (1.9 mg) [0.1 mg/kg: 1st dose]   1.3 mL (3.8 mg) [0.2 mg/kg: 2nd dose]
concentration: 6 mg/2 mL

Amiodarone: 1.9 mL (95 mg)
[V-Tach with Pulse: Mix 1.9 mL in 100 mL NS: 50 drops/min; 10 drop set] [5 mg/kg]
concentration: 150 mg/ 3 mL

Atropine: 3.8 mL (0.38 mg) [0.02 mg/kg] concentration: 1 mg/10 mL

Benadryl: 0.4 mL (19 mg) [1 mg/kg] concentration: 50 mg/mL

Calcium Chloride: Mix 3.8 mL (380 mg) in 6 mL NS; Slow IV/IO [20 mg/kg]
concentration: 1000 mg/10 mL

Dextrose 25%: Mix 19 mL D50W + 19 mL NS (9.5 G) [0.5 G/kg] concentration: 1 G/2 mL

Dopamine: Mix 10 mL Dopamine + 100 mL NS: 36 drops/min. [5 mcg/kg/min]
concentration: 16,000 mcg/100 mL

Epinephrine 1:10,000: 1.9 mL (0.19 mg) [0.01 mg/kg]   concentration: 1 mg/10 mL

Epinephrine 1:1000: ET: Mix 1.9 mL Epi 1:1000 + 1.1 mL NS (1.9 mg) [0.1 mg/kg]
concentration: 1 mg/mL

Epinephrine 1:1000: SQ/IM: 0.2 mL (0.2 mg)   Epi-Pen Jr. (0.15 mg)

Epinephrine: Nebulized: 5 mL Epi 1:1000 (0.5 mg)

Fentanyl: 0.4 mL (19 mcg) [1 mcg/kg] concentration: 50 mcg/mL

Fluid Bolus: 380 mL

Glucagon: 1 mL (1 mg)   [0.1 mg/kg] concentration: 1 mg/mL

Ibuprofen: 9.5 mL (190 mg) [10 mg/kg] concentration: 20 mg/mL

Lidocaine: 1 mL (19 mg) [1 mg/kg] concentration: 100 mg/5 mL

Magnesium Sulfate:
concentration: 1 G/2 mL: Mix 1.9 mL (950 mg) Mag Sulfate + 100 mL NS: 100 drops/min.; 10 drop set
concentration: 2 G/50 mL: Mix 23.8 mL (950 mg) Mag Sulfate + 100 mL NS: 100 drops/min.;10 drop set
[50 mg/kg]

4 y/o   19 kg

Morphine: Mix 5 mg/mL Morphine in 9 mL NS: 3.8 mL (1.9 mg)   [0.1 mg/kg]
concentration: 1 mg/2mL

Narcan: 1.9 mL (1.9 mg)   [0.1 mg/kg]   concentration 1 mg/mL

Sodium Bicarbonate: 19 mL (19 mEq)   [1 mEq/kg]   concentration 1 mEq/mL

Solumedrol: 0.6 mL (38 mg) [2 mg/kg] concentration 62.5 mg/mL

Valium:
IV/IO: 0.8 mL (3.8 mg) [0.2 mg/kg]
Rectal: 1.5 mL (7.6 mg) [0.4 mg/kg]
concentration: 5 mg/mL

Versed:
concentration: 1 mg/mL: 3.8 mL (3.8 mg) [0.2 mg/kg]
concentration: 5 mg/mL: 0.8 mL (3.8 mg) [0.2 mg/kg]

Zofran: Mix 1 mL (1.9 mg) in 2 mL NS, Slow IVP   [0.1 mg/kg]   concentration: 2 mg/mL

BVM: Tidal volume: 133 mL

ETT: 5.0 – 5.5   Depth: 15 cm

 Supraglottic Airway: #2   OPA: 70 mm (White)   NPA: 24 F

Cardioversion: #1: 19 J #2: 38 J

 Defibrillation: #1: 38 J #2: 76 J #3: 114 J #4: 152 J #5: 190 J

*" The LORD gives me light and saves me. Why should I fear anyone? The LORD is my place of safety.
Why should I be afraid."   -Psalm 27:1*

5 y/o   22 kg   (Blue)

Acetaminophen: 10.3 mL (330 mg) [15 mg/kg]   concentration: 160 mg/5 mL

Adenosine: 0.7 mL (2.2 mg) [0.1 mg/kg: 1st dose]   1.5 mL (4.4 mg) [0.2 mg/kg: 2nd dose]
concentration: 6 mg/2 mL

Amiodarone: 2.2 mL (110mg)
[V-Tach with Pulse: Mix 2.2 mL in 100 mL NS: 50 drops/min; 10 drop set]   [5 mg/kg]
concentration: 150 mg/ 3 mL

Atropine: 4.4 mL (0.44 mg)   [0.02 mg/kg] concentration: 1 mg/10 mL

Benadryl: 0.4 mL (22 mg) [1 mg/kg] concentration: 50 mg/mL

Calcium Chloride: Mix 4.4 mL (440 mg) in 5 mL NS; Slow IV/IO [20 mg/kg]
concentration: 1000 mg/10 mL

Dextrose 25%: Mix 22 mL D50W + 22 mL NS (11 G) [0.5 G/kg] concentration: 1 G/2 mL

Dopamine: Mix 10 mL Dopamine + 100 mL NS: 41 drops/min. [5 mcg/kg/min]
concentration: 16,000 mcg/100 mL

Epinephrine 1:10,000: 2.2 mL (0.22 mg) [0.01 mg/kg]   concentration: 1 mg/10 mL

Epinephrine 1:1000: ET: Mix 2.2 mL Epi 1:1000 + 0.8 mL NS (2.2 mg) [0.1 mg/kg]
concentration: 1 mg/mL

Epinephrine 1:1000: SQ/IM: 0.2 mL (0.2 mg)   Epi-Pen Jr. (0.15 mg)

Epinephrine: Nebulized: 5 mL Epi 1:1000 (0.5 mg)

Fentanyl: 0.4 mL (22 mcg) [1 mcg/kg] concentration: 50 mcg/mL

Fluid Bolus: 440 mL

Glucagon: 1 mL (1 mg)   [0.1 mg/kg] concentration: 1 mg/mL

Ibuprofen: 11 mL (220 mg) [10 mg/kg] concentration: 20 mg/mL

Lidocaine: 1.1 mL (22 mg) [1 mg/kg] concentration: 100 mg/5 mL

Magnesium Sulfate:
concentration: 1 G/2 mL: Mix 2.2 mL (1100 mg) Mag Sulfate + 100 mL NS: 100 drops/min.; 10 drop set
concentration: 2 G/50 mL: Mix 27.5 mL(1100 mg) Mag Sulfate + 100 mL NS:100 drops/min.;10 drop set
[50 mg/kg]

5 y/o   22 kg

Morphine: Mix 5 mg/mL Morphine in 9 mL NS: 4.4 mL (2.2 mg)   [0.1 mg/kg]
concentration: 1 mg/2mL

Narcan: 2 mL (2 mg)   [0.1 mg/kg] concentration 1 mg/mL

Sodium Bicarbonate: 22 mL (22 mEq)   [1 mEq/kg]   concentration 1 mEq/mL

Solumedrol: 0.7 mL (44 mg)   [2 mg/kg]   concentration 62.5 mg/mL

Valium:
IV/IO: 0.9 mL (4.4 mg) [0.2 mg/kg]
Rectal: 1.8 mL (8.8 mg) [0.4 mg/kg]
concentration: 5 mg/mL

Versed:
concentration: 1 mg/mL: 4.4 mL (4.4 mg) [0.2 mg/kg]
concentration: 5 mg/mL: 0.9 mL (4.4 mg) [0.2 mg/kg]

Zofran: Mix 1.1 mL (2.2 mg) in 2 mL NS, Slow IVP   [0.1 mg/kg]   concentration: 2 mg/mL

BVM: Tidal volume: 154 mL

ETT: 5.0 – 5.5   Depth: 15.5 cm

Supraglottic Airway: #2.5   OPA: 70 mm (White)   NPA: 24 F

Cardioversion: #1: 22J   #2: 44 J

Defibrillation: #1: 44 J   #2: 88 J   #3: 132 J   #4: 176 J   #5: 220 J

"Don't just talk about love; put your love into action."   1 John 3:18

Acetaminophen: 11.7 mL (375 mg) [15 mg/kg] concentration: 160 mg/5 mL

Adenosine: 0.8 mL (2.5 mg) [0.1 mg/kg: 1st dose]   1.7 mL (5 mg) [0.2 mg/kg: 2nd dose] concentration: 6 mg/2 mL

Amiodarone: 2.5 mL (125 mg)
[V-Tach with Pulse: Mix 2.5 mL in 100 mL NS: 50 drops/min; 10 drop set] [5 mg/kg]
concentration: 150 mg/ 3 mL

Atropine: 5 mL (0.5 mg) [0.02 mg/kg] concentration: 1 mg/10 mL

Benadryl: 0.5 mL (25 mg) [1 mg/kg] concentration: 50 mg/mL

Calcium Chloride: Mix 5 mL (500 mg)in 5 mL NS; Slow IV/IO [20 mg/kg]
concentration: 1000 mg/10 mL

Dextrose 25%: Mix 25 mL D50W + 25 mL NS (12.5 G) [0.5 G/kg] concentration: 1 G/2 mL

Dopamine: Mix 10 mL Dopamine + 100 mL NS: 47 drops/min. [5 mcg/kg/min]
concentration: 16,000 mcg/100 mL

Epinephrine 1:10,000: 2.5 mL (0.25 mg) [0.01 mg/kg] concentration: 1 mg/10 mL

Epinephrine 1:1000: ET: Mix 2.5 mL Epi 1:1000 + 0.5 mL NS (2.5 mg) [0.1 mg/kg]
concentration: 1 mg/mL

Epinephrine 1:1000: SQ/IM: 0.2 mL (0.2 mg)   Epi-Pen Jr. (0.15 mg)

Epinephrine: Nebulized: 5 mL Epi 1:1000 (0.5 mg)

Fentanyl: 0.5 mL (25 mcg) [1 mcg/kg] concentration: 50 mcg/mL

Fluid Bolus: 500 mL

Glucagon: 1 mL (1 mg)   [0.1 mg/kg] concentration: 1 mg/mL

Haldol: 0.8 mL (3.8 mg) IM only   [0.15 mg/kg]   concentration: 5 mg/mL

Ibuprofen: 12.5 mL (250 mg) [10 mg/kg]   concentration: 20 mg/mL

Lidocaine: 1.3 mL (25 mg) [1 mg/kg] concentration: 100 mg/5 mL

Magnesium Sulfate:
concentration: 1 G/2 mL: Mix 2.5 mL (1250 mg) Mag Sulfate + 100 mL NS: 100 drops/min.; 10 drop set
concentration: 2 G/50 mL: Mix 31.3 mL(1250 mg) Mag Sulfate + 100 mL NS:100 drops/min.;10 drop set
[50 mg/kg]

6 y/o   25 kg

Morphine: Mix 5 mg/mL Morphine in 9 mL NS: 5 mL (2.5 mg)   [0.1 mg/kg]
concentration: 1 mg/2mL

Narcan: 2 mL (2 mg)   [0.1 mg/kg]   concentration 1 mg/mL

Sodium Bicarbonate: 25 mL (25 mEq)   [1 mEq/kg]   concentration 1 mEq/mL

Solumedrol: 0.8 mL (50 mg)   [2 mg/kg]   concentration 62.5 mg/mL

Valium:
IV/IO: 1 mL (5 mg) [0.2 mg/kg]
Rectal: 2 mL (10 mg) [0.4 mg/kg]
concentration: 5 mg/mL

Versed:
concentration: 1 mg/mL: 5 mL (5 mg) [0.2 mg/kg]
concentration: 5 mg/mL: 1 mL (5 mg) [0.2 mg/kg]

Zofran: Mix 1.3 mL (2.5 mg) in 2 mL NS, Slow IVP   [0.1 mg/kg]   concentration: 2 mg/mL

BVM: Tidal volume: 175 mL

ETT: 5.0 -5.5   Depth: 16 cm

Supraglottic Airway: #2.5   OPA: 80 mm (Green)   NPA: 26 F

Cardioversion: #1: 25 J #2: 50 J

Defibrillation: #1: 50 J #2: 100 J #3: 150 J #4: 200 J #5: 250 J

"The LORD of heaven and earth, has hidden these things from the wise and learned, and revealed them to little children." ---Luke 10:21

Acetaminophen: 13.1 mL (420 mg) [15 mg/kg]   concentration: 160 mg/5 mL

Adenosine: 0.9 mL (2.8 mg) [0.1 mg/kg: 1st dose]   1.9 mL (5.6 mg) [0.2 mg/kg: 2nd dose]
concentration: 6 mg/2 mL

Amiodarone: 2.8 mL (140 mg)
[V-Tach with Pulse: Mix 2.8 mL in 100 mL NS: 50 drops/min;10 drop set] [5 mg/kg]
concentration: 150 mg/ 3 mL

Atropine: 5 mL (0.5 mg) [0.02 mg/kg] concentration: 1 mg/10 mL

Benadryl: 0.6 mL (28 mg) [1 mg/kg]   concentration: 50 mg/mL

Calcium Chloride: Mix 5.6 mL (560 mg) in 4 mL NS; Slow IV/IO [20 mg/kg]
concentration: 1000 mg/10 mL

Dextrose 25%: Mix 28 mL D50W + 28 mL NS (14 G) [0.5 G/kg] concentration: 1 G/2 mL

Dopamine: Mix 10 mL Dopamine + 100 mL NS: 53 drops/min. [5 mcg/kg/min]
concentration: 16,000 mcg/100 mL

Epinephrine 1:10,000: 2.8 mL (0.28 mg) [0.01 mg/kg]   concentration: 1 mg/10 mL

Epinephrine 1:1000: ET: Mix 2.8 mL Epi 1:1000 + 0.2 mL NS (2.8 mg)   [0.1 mg/kg]
concentration: 1 mg/mL

Epinephrine 1:1000: SQ/IM: 0.2 mL (0.2 mg)   Epi-Pen Jr. (0.15 mg)

Epinephrine: Nebulized: 5 mL Epi 1:1000 (0.5 mg)

Fentanyl: 0.6 mL (28 mcg) [1 mcg/kg] concentration: 50 mcg/mL

Fluid Bolus: 560 mL

Glucagon: 1 mL (1 mg)   [0.1 mg/kg] concentration: 1 mg/mL

Haldol: 0.8 mL (4.2 mg) IM only   [0.15 mg/kg]   concentration 5 mg/mL

Ibuprofen: 14 mL (280 mg)   [10 mg/kg]   concentration: 20 mg/mL

Lidocaine: 1.4 mL (28 mg) [1 mg/kg] concentration: 100 mg/5 mL

Magnesium Sulfate:
concentration: 1 G/2 mL: Mix 2.8 mL (1400 mg) Mag Sulfate + 100 mL NS: 100 drops/min.; 10 drop set
concentration: 2 G/50 mL: Mix 35 mL (1400 mg) Mag Sulfate + 100 mL NS: 100 drops/min.; 10 drop set
[50 mg/kg]

7 y/o   28 kg

Morphine: Mix 5 mg/mL Morphine in 9 mL NS: 5.6 mL (2.8 mg)   [0.1 mg/kg]
concentration: 1 mg/2mL

Narcan: 2 mL (2 mg)   [0.1 mg/kg]   concentration 1 mg/mL

Sodium Bicarbonate: 28 mL (28 mEq)   [1 mEq/kg]   concentration 1 mEq/mL

Solumedrol: 0.9 mL (56 mg)   [2 mg/kg]   concentration 62.5 mg/mL

Valium:
IV/IO: 1 mL (5.6 mg) [0.2 mg/kg]
Rectal: 2 mL (10 mg) [0.4 mg/kg]
concentration: 5 mg/mL

Versed:
concentration: 1 mg/mL: 5 mL (5 mg) [0.2 mg/kg]
concentration: 5 mg/mL: 1 mL (5 mg) [0.2 mg/kg]

Zofran: Mix 1.4 mL (2.8 mg) in 2 mL NS, Slow IVP   [0.1 mg/kg]   concentration: 2 mg/mL

BVM: Tidal volume: 196 mL

ETT: 5.0 – 6.0   Depth: 16.5 cm

Supraglottic Airway: #2.5   OPA: 80 mm (Green)   NPA: 26 F

Cardioversion: #1: 28 J #2: 56 J

Defibrillation: #1: 56 J #2: 112 J #3: 168 J #4: 224 J #5: 280 J

" When you enter a town, heal the sick people who are there."   - Luke 10:8-9

8 y/o   31 kg   (Green)

Acetaminophen: 14.5 mL (465 mg) [15 mg/kg] concentration: 160 mg/5 mL

Adenosine: 1 mL (3.1 mg) [0.1 mg/kg: 1st dose]   2.1 mL (6.2 mg) [0.2 mg/kg: 2nd dose]
concentration: 6 mg/2 mL

Amiodarone: 3.1 mL (155 mg)
[V-Tach with Pulse: Mix 3 mL in 100 mL NS: 50 drops/min; 10 drop set] [5 mg/kg]
concentration: 150 mg/ 3 mL

Atropine: 5 mL (0.5 mg) [0.02 mg/kg] concentration: 1 mg/10 mL

Benadryl: 0.6 mL (31 mg) [1 mg/kg] concentration: 50 mg/mL

Calcium Chloride: Mix 6.2 mL (620 mg) in 3 mL NS; Slow IV/IO [20 mg/kg]
concentration: 1000 mg/10 mL

Dextrose 25%: Mix 31 mL D50W + 31 mL NS (15.5 G) [0.5 G/kg] concentration: 1 G/2 mL

Dopamine: Mix 10 mL Dopamine + 100 mL NS: 58 drops/min. [5 mcg/kg/min]
concentration: 16,000 mcg/100 mL

Epinephrine 1:10,000: 3.1 mL (0.31 mg) [0.01 mg/kg] concentration: 1 mg/10 mL

Epinephrine 1:1000: ET: 3.1 mL (3.1 mg) [0.1 mg/kg] concentration: 1 mg/mL

Epinephrine 1:1000: SQ/IM: 0.2 mL (0.2 mg)   Epi-Pen (0.3 mg)

Epinephrine: Nebulized: 5 mL Epi 1:1000 (0.5 mg)

Fentanyl: 0.6 mL (31 mcg) [1 mcg/kg] concentration: 50 mcg/mL

Fluid Bolus: 620 mL

Glucagon: 1 mL (1 mg)   [0.1 mg/kg] concentration: 1 mg/mL

Haldol: 0.9 mL (4.7 mg) IM Only [0.15 mg/kg] concentration: 5 mg/mL

Ibuprofen: 15.5 mL (310 mg) [10 mg/kg] concentration 20 mg/mL

Lidocaine: 1.6 mL (31 mg) [1 mg/kg] concentration: 100 mg/5 mL

Magnesium Sulfate:
concentration: 1 G/2 mL: Mix 3.1 mL (1550 mg) Mag Sulfate + 100 mL NS: 100 drops/min.; 10 drop set
concentration: 2 G/50 mL: Mix 38.8 mL(1550 mg) Mag Sulfate + 100 mL NS:100 drops/min.;10 drop set
[50 mg/kg]

8 y/o   31 kg

Morphine: Mix 5 mg/mL Morphine in 9 mL NS: 6.2 mL (3.1 mg)   [0.1 mg/kg]
concentration: 1 mg/2mL

Narcan: 2 mL (2 mg)   [0.1 mg/kg]   concentration 1 mg/mL

Sodium Bicarbonate: 31 mL (31 mEq)   [1 mEq/kg]   concentration 1 mEq/mL

Solumedrol: 1 mL (62 mg)   [2 mg/kg]   concentration 62.5 mg/mL

Valium:
IV/IO: 1.2 mL (6.2 mg) [0.2 mg/kg]
Rectal: 2.5 mL (12.4 mg) [0.4 mg/kg]
concentration: 5 mg/mL

Versed:
concentration: 1 mg/mL: 5 mL (5 mg) [0.2 mg/kg]
concentration: 5 mg/mL: 1 mL (5 mg) [0.2 mg/kg]

Zofran: Mix 1.6 mL (3.1 mg) in 2 mL NS, Slow IVP   [0.1 mg/kg]   concentration: 2 mg/mL

BVM: Tidal volume: 217 mL

ETT: 6.0   Depth: 17 cm

Supraglottic Airway: #3   OPA: 80 mm (Green)   NPA: 26 F

Cardioversion: #1: 31 J #2: 62 J

Defibrillation: #1: 62 J #2: 124 J #3: 186 J #4: 248 J #5: 310 J

"Even though I walk through the valley of the shadow of death, I will have no fear. God is with me." -
Psalm 23:4

9 y/o   34 kg   (Green)

Acetaminophen: 15.9 mL (510 mg) [15 mg/kg]   concentration: 160 mg/5 mL

Adenosine: 1.1 mL (3.4 mg) [0.1 mg/kg: 1st dose]   2.3 mL (6.8 mg) [0.2 mg/kg: 2nd dose]
concentration: 6 mg/2 mL

Amiodarone: 3.4 mL (170 mg)
[V-Tach with Pulse: Mix 3 mL in 100 mL NS: 50 drops/min; 10 drop set]   [5 mg/kg]
concentration: 150 mg/ 3 mL

Atropine: 5 mL (0.5 mg) [0.02 mg/kg] concentration: 1 mg/10 mL

Benadryl: 0.7 mL (34 mg) [1 mg/kg] concentration: 50 mg/mL

Calcium Chloride: Mix 6.8 mL (680 mg) in 3 mL NS; Slow IV/IO [20 mg/kg]
concentration: 1000 mg/10 mL

Dextrose 25%: Mix 34 mL D50W + 34 mL NS (17 G) [0.5 G/kg] concentration: 1 G/2 mL

Dopamine: Mix 10 mL Dopamine + 100 mL NS: 64 drops/min. [5 mcg/kg/min]
concentration: 16,000 mcg/100 mL

Epinephrine 1:10,000: 3.4 mL (0.34 mg) [0.01 mg/kg]   concentration: 1 mg/10 mL

Epinephrine 1:1000: ET: 3.4 mL (3.4 mg) [0.1 mg/kg] concentration: 1 mg/mL

Epinephrine 1:1000: SQ/IM: 0.3 mL (0.3 mg)   Epi-Pen (0.3 mg)

Epinephrine: Nebulized: 5 mL Epi 1:1000 (5 mg)

Fentanyl: 0.7 mL (34 mcg) [1 mcg/kg] concentration: 50 mcg/mL

Fluid Bolus: 680 mL

Glucagon: 1 mL (1 mg)   [0.1 mg/kg] concentration: 1 mg/mL

Haldol: 1 mL (5 mg) IM Only   [0.15 mg/kg]   concentration: 5 mg/mL

Ibuprofen: 17 mL (340 mg) [10 mg/kg] concentration 20 mg/mL

Lidocaine: 1.7 mL (34 mg) [1 mg/kg] concentration: 100 mg/5 mL

Magnesium Sulfate:
concentration: 1 G/2 mL: Mix 3.4 mL (1700 mg) Mag Sulfate + 100 mL NS: 100 drops/min.; 10 drop set
concentration: 2 G/50 mL: Mix 42.5 mL(1700 mg) Mag Sulfate + 100 mL NS:100 drops/min.;10 drop set
[50 mg/kg]

9 y/o   34 kg

Morphine: Mix 5 mg/mL Morphine in 9 mL NS: 6.8 mL (3.4 mg)   [0.1 mg/kg]
concentration: 1 mg/2mL

Narcan: 2 mL (2 mg)   [0.1 mg/kg] concentration 1 mg/mL

Sodium Bicarbonate: 34 mL (34 mEq)   [1 mEq/kg]   concentration 1 mEq/mL

Solumedrol: 1.1 mL (68 mg)   [2 mg/kg]   concentration 62.5 mg/mL

Valium:
IV/IO: 1.4 mL (6.8 mg) [0.2 mg/kg]
Rectal: 2 mL (10 mg) [0.4 mg/kg]
concentration: 5 mg/mL

Versed:
concentration: 1 mg/mL: 5 mL (5 mg) [0.2 mg/kg]
concentration: 5 mg/mL: 1 mL (5 mg) [0.2 mg/kg]

Zofran: Mix 1.7 mL (3.4 mg) in 2 mL NS, Slow IVP   [0.1 mg/kg]   concentration: 2 mg/mL

BVM: Tidal volume: 238 mL

ETT: 6.0   Depth: 17.5 cm

Supraglottic Airway: #3   OPA: 80 mm (Green)   NPA: 26 F

Cardioversion: #1: 34 J #2: 68 J

 Defibrillation: #1: 68 J #2: 136 J #3: 204 J #4: 272 J #5: 340 J

" In all things God works for the good of those who love Him and are called according to His purpose."
-Romans 8:28

Acetaminophen: 17.3 mL (555 mg) [15 mg/kg] concentration: 160 mg/5 mL

Adenosine: 1.2 mL (3.7 mg) [0.1 mg/kg: 1st dose]   2.5 mL (7.4 mg) [0.2 mg/kg: 2nd dose] concentration: 6 mg/2 mL

Amiodarone: 3.7 mL (185 mg)
[V-Tach with Pulse: Mix 3 mL in 100 mL NS; 50 drops/min; 10 drop set]   [5 mg/kg]
concentration: 150 mg/ 3 mL

Atropine: 5 mL (0.5 mg) [0.02 mg/kg] concentration: 1 mg/10 mL

Benadryl: 0.7 mL (37 mg) [1 mg/kg] concentration: 50 mg/mL

Calcium Chloride: Mix 7.4 mL (740 mg) in 2 mL NS; Slow IV/IO [20 mg/kg]
concentration: 1000 mg/10 mL

Dextrose 25%: Mix 37 mL D50W + 37 mL NS (18.5 G) [0.5 G/kg] concentration: 1 G/2 mL

Dopamine: Mix 10 mL Dopamine + 100 mL NS: 69 drops/min. [5 mcg/kg/min]
concentration: 16,000 mcg/100 mL

Epinephrine 1:10,000: 3.7 mL (0.37 mg) [0.01 mg/kg] concentration: 1 mg/10 mL

Epinephrine 1:1000: ET: 3.7 mL (3.7 mg) [0.1 mg/kg] concentration: 1 mg/mL

Epinephrine 1:1000: SQ/IM: 0.3 mL (0.3 mg)   Epi-Pen Jr. (0.3 mg)

Epinephrine: Nebulized: 5 mL Epi 1:1000 (0.5 mg)

Fentanyl: 0.7 mL (37 mcg) [1 mcg/kg] concentration: 50 mcg/mL

Fluid Bolus: 740 mL

Glucagon: 1 mL (1 mg)   [0.1 mg/kg] concentration: 1 mg/mL

Haldol: 1 mL (5 mg) IM Only   [0.15 mg/kg]   concentration: 5 mg/mL

Ibuprofen: 18.5 mL (370 mg) [10 mg/kg] concentration 20 mg/mL

Lidocaine: 1.9 mL (37 mg) [1 mg/kg] concentration: 100 mg/5 mL

Magnesium Sulfate:
concentration: 1 G/2 mL: Mix 3.7 mL (1850 mg) Mag Sulfate + 100 mL NS: 100 drops/min.; 10 drop set
concentration: 2 G/50 mL: Mix 46.3 mL(1850 mg) Mag Sulfate + 100 mL NS:100 drops/min.;10 drop set
[50 mg/kg]

10 y/o   37 kg

Morphine: Mix 5 mg/mL Morphine in 9 mL NS: 7.4 mL (3.7 mg)   [0.1 mg/kg]
concentration: 1 mg/2mL

Narcan: 2 mL (2 mg)   [0.1 mg/kg]   concentration 1 mg/mL

Sodium Bicarbonate: 37 mL (37 mEq)   [1 mEq/kg]   concentration 1 mEq/mL

Solumedrol: 1.2 mL (74 mg)   [2 mg/kg]   concentration 62.5 mg/mL

Valium:
IV/IO: 1.5 mL (7.4 mg) [0.2 mg/kg]
Rectal: 2 mL (10 mg) [0.4 mg/kg]
concentration: 5 mg/mL

Versed:
concentration: 1 mg/mL: 5 mL (5 mg) [0.2 mg/kg]
concentration: 5 mg/mL: 1 mL (5 mg) [0.2 mg/kg]

Zofran: Mix 1.9 mL (3.7 mg) in 2 mL NS, Slow IVP   [0.1 mg/kg]   concentration: 2 mg/mL

BVM: Tidal volume: 259 mL

ETT: 6.5   Depth: 18 cm

Supraglottic Airway: #3   OPA: 80 mm (Green)   NPA: 26 - 28 F

Cardioversion: #1: 37 J #2: 74 J

Defibrillation: #1: 74 J #2: 148 J #3: 222 J #4: 296 J #5: 360 J

" Let your light shine in front of others. They will see the good things you do and they will praise your Father in heaven." -Matthew 5:16

11 y/o   40 kg

Acetaminophen: 18.8 mL (600 mg) [15 mg/kg]   concentration: 160 mg/5 mL

Adenosine: 1.3 mL (4 mg) [0.1 mg/kg: 1st dose]   2.7 mL (8 mg) [0.2 mg/kg: 2nd dose]
concentration: 6 mg/2 mL

Amiodarone: 4 mL (200 mg)
[V-Tach with Pulse: Mix 3 mL in 100 mL NS: 50 drops/min; 10 drop set] [5 mg/kg]
concentration: 150 mg/ 3 mL

Atropine: 5 mL (0.5 mg) [0.02 mg/kg] concentration: 1 mg/10 mL

Benadryl: 0.8 mL (40 mg) [1 mg/kg]   concentration: 50 mg/mL

Calcium Chloride: Mix 8 mL (800 mg) in 2 mL NS; Slow IV/IO [20 mg/kg]
concentration: 1000 mg/10 mL

Dextrose 25%: Mix 40 mL D50W + 40 mL NS (20 G) [0.5 G/kg] concentration: 1 G/2 mL

Dopamine: Mix 10 mL Dopamine + 100 mL NS: 75 drops/min. [5 mcg/kg/min]
concentration: 16,000 mcg/100 mL

Epinephrine 1:10,000: 4 mL (0.4 mg) [0.01 mg/kg]   concentration: 1 mg/10 mL

Epinephrine 1:1000: ET: 4 mL (4 mg) [0.1 mg/kg] concentration: 1 mg/mL

Epinephrine 1:1000: SQ/IM: 0.3 mL (0.3 mg)   Epi-Pen (0.3 mg)

Epinephrine: Nebulized: 5 mL Epi 1:1000 (5 mg)

Fentanyl: 0.8 mL (40 mcg) [1 mcg/kg]   concentration: 50 mcg/mL

Fluid Bolus: 800 mL

Glucagon: 1 mL (1 mg)   [0.1 mg/kg] concentration: 1 mg/mL

Haldol: 1 mL (5 mg) IM Only [0.15 mg/kg] concentration: 5 mg/mL

Ibuprofen: 20 mL (400 mg) [10 mg/kg] concentration 20 mg/mL

Lidocaine: 2 mL (40 mg) [1 mg/kg] concentration: 100 mg/5 mL

Magnesium Sulfate:
concentration: 1 G/2 mL: Mix 4 mL (2000 mg) Mag Sulfate + 100 mL NS: 100 drops/min.; 10 drop set
concentration: 2 G/50 mL: 50 drops/min.; 10 drop set [50 mg/kg]

Morphine: Mix 5 mg/mL Morphine in 9 mL NS: 8 mL (4 mg)   [0.1 mg/kg]
concentration: 1 mg/2mL

11 y/o   40 kg

Narcan: 2 mL (2 mg)   [0.1 mg/kg]   concentration 1 mg/mL

Sodium Bicarbonate: 40 mL (40 mEq)   [1 mEq/kg]   concentration 1 mEq/mL

Solumedrol: 1.3 mL (80 mg)   [2 mg/kg]   concentration 62.5 mg/mL

Valium:
IV/IO: 1.6 mL (8 mg) [0.2 mg/kg]
Rectal: 2 mL (10 mg) [0.4 mg/kg]
concentration: 5 mg/mL

Versed:
concentration: 1 mg/mL: 5 mL (5 mg) [0.2 mg/kg]
concentration: 5 mg/mL: 1 mL (5 mg) [0.2 mg/kg]

Zofran: Mix 2 mL (4 mg) Zofran + 2 mL NS: Slow IVP   [0.1 mg/kg]   concentration: 2 mg/mL

BVM: Tidal volume: 280 mL

ETT: 6.5   Depth: 18.5 cm

Supraglottic Airway: #3   OPA: 80 mm (Green)   NPA: 28 F

Cardioversion: #1: 40 J #2: 80 J

Defibrillation: #1: 80 J #2: 160 J #3: 240 J #4: 320 J #5: 360 J

" God demonstrates His love for us in this: while we were still sinners, Christ died for us."
Romans 5:8

12-14 y/o   43-50 kg

Acetaminophen: 20.2-23.4 mL (645-750 mg) [15 mg/kg]   concentration: 160 mg/5 mL

Adenosine:
1.4 -1.7 mL(4.3-5 mg) [0.1 mg/kg: 1st dose]
2.9 -3.3 mL (8.6-10 mg) [0.2 mg/kg: 2nd dose]
concentration 6 mg/2 mL

Amiodarone: 4.3-5 mL(215-250 mg)
[V-Tach with Pulse: Mix 3 mL in 100 mL NS:50 drops/min;10 drop set [5mg/kg]
concentration:150 mg/ 3 mL

Atropine: 5 mL (0.5 mg) [0.02 mg/kg] concentration: 1 mg/10 mL

Benadryl: 0.9-1 mL (43-50 mg) [1 mg/kg]   concentration: 50 mg/mL

Calcium Chloride: Mix 8.6- 10 mL (860- 1000 mg) ; Slow IV/IO [20 mg/kg]
concentration: 1000 mg/10 mL

Dextrose 25%: Mix 43- 50 mL D50W + 43- 50 mL NS (21.5- 25 G) [0.5 G/kg] concentration: 1 G/2 mL

Dopamine: Mix 10 mL Dopamine + 100 mL NS: 81- 94 drops/min. [5 mcg/kg/min]
concentration: 16,000 mcg/100 mL

Epinephrine 1:10,000: 4.3- 5 mL (0.43-0.5 mg) [0.01 mg/kg]   concentration: 1 mg/10 mL

Epinephrine 1:1000: ET: 4.3- 5 mL (4.3- 5 mg) [0.1 mg/kg] concentration: 1 mg/mL

Epinephrine 1:1000: SQ/IM: 0.3 mL (0.3 mg)   Epi-Pen (0.3 mg)

Epinephrine: Nebulized: 5 mL Epi 1:1000 (5 mg)

Fentanyl: 0.9-1 mL (43-50 mcg) [1 mcg/kg]   concentration: 50 mcg/mL

Fluid Bolus: 860-1000 mL

Glucagon: 1 mL (1 mg)   [0.1 mg/kg] concentration: 1 mg/mL

Haldol: 1 mL (5 mg) IM Only [0.15 mg/kg] concentration: 5 mg/mL

Ibuprofen: 21.5- 25 mL (430- 500 mg) [10 mg/kg] concentration 20 mg/mL

Lidocaine: 2.2- 2.5 mL (43-50 mg) [1 mg/kg] concentration: 100 mg/5 mL

Magnesium Sulfate:
concentration: 1 G/2 mL: Mix 4 mL (2000 mg) Mag Sulfate + 100 mL NS: 100 drops/min.; 10 drop set
concentration: 2 G/50 mL: 50 drops/min.; 10 drop set [50 mg/kg]

12-14 y/o   43-50 kg

Morphine: Mix 5 mg/mL Morphine in 9 mL NS: 8.6-10 mL (4.3- 5 mg)   [0.1 mg/kg]
concentration: 1 mg/2mL

Narcan: 2 mL (2 mg)   [0.1 mg/kg]   concentration 1 mg/mL

Sodium Bicarbonate: 43-50 mL (43-50 mEq)   [1 mEq/kg]   concentration 1 mEq/mL

Solumedrol: 1.3 mL (80 mg)   [2 mg/kg]   concentration 62.5 mg/mL

Valium:
IV/IO: 1.7-2 mL (8.6- 10 mg) [0.2 mg/kg]
Rectal: 2 mL (10 mg) [0.4 mg/kg]
concentration: 5 mg/mL

Versed:
concentration: 1 mg/mL: 5 mL (5 mg) [0.2 mg/kg]
concentration: 5 mg/mL: 1 mL (5 mg) [0.2 mg/kg]

Zofran: Mix 2 mL (4 mg) Zofran + 2 mL NS: Slow IVP   [0.1 mg/kg]   concentration: 2 mg/mL

BVM:Tidal volume: 301-350 mL

ETT: 6.5- 7.0   Depth: 19-20 cm

Supraglottic Airway: #3-#4   OPA: 80-90mm (Green/Yellow)   NPA:28-30 F

Cardioversion: #1: 43-50 J #2: 86-100 J

 Defibrillation: #1: 86-100 J #2: 172-200 J #3: 258-300 J #4: 344-360 J #5: 360 J

 " For God so loved the world, He gave His only begotten Son, that whoever believes in Him shall not die, but have eternal life." -John 3:16

APGAR	0	1	2
Appearance	Body: Cyanosis Extremities: Cyanosis	Body: Normal Extremities: Cyanosis	Body: Normal Extremities: Normal
Pulse	Absent	<100	>100
Grimace	None	Grimace, Flinch	Coughs, Cries
Activity	Limp	Flexion of Extremities	Active Motion
Respirations	Absent	Slow, Irregular	Strong Cry, Normal

Pediatric Glasgow Coma Scale

Eye Opening	>1 y/o	<1 y/o	
	Spontaneous	Spontaneous	4
	To Speech	To Speech	3
	To Pain	To Pain	2
	None	None	1

Verbal	>5 y/o	2-5 y/o	0-2 y/o	
	Oriented	Appropriate Words/ Phrases	Smiles, Coos	5
	Disoriented/Confused	Inappropriate Words/Phrases	Inconsolable Crying	4
	Inappropriate Words	Crying/Screaming	Crying/Screaming	3
	Incomprehensible Sounds	Grunts	Grunts/Agitated/ Restless	2
	None	None	None	1

Motor	>1 y/o	<1 y/o	
	Obeys	Spontaneous	6
	Localizes Pain	Localizes Pain	5
	Withdrawal	Withdrawal	4
	Flexion-Decorticate	Flexion-Decorticate	3
	Extension-Decerebrate	Extension-Decerebrate	2
	None	None	1

Pediatric Vital Signs

Age	Pulse	Respirations	Blood Pressure	Hypotensive
Newborn to 1 m/o	140-150	40-60	60 + age in months	<60/systolic
1 m/o to 1 y/o	130-140	30-40	70 + (age x 2)	<70 + (age x 2)
1 y/o to 4 y/o	120-130	20-30	80 + (age x 2)	<70 + (age x 2)
4 y/o to 8 y/o	100-120	20-30	80 + (age x 2)	<70 + (age x 2)
8 y/o to 10 y/o	80-100	12-20	80 + (age x 2)	<70 + (age x 2)
10 y/o-18 y/o	80-100	12-20	90 + (age x 2)	<90/systolic

Pediatric Trauma Score

	+ 2	+ 1	-1
Weight (kg)	>20	10-20	< 10
Airway	Patent	Maintainable	Non-Maintainable
Systolic B/P	>90	50-90	< 50
Mental Status	Awake	Altered	Unresponsive
Open Wound/Bleeding	None	Minor	Major
Extremity Fracture	None	Closed/Singular	Open or Multiple

Age Estimation Formula: >1 y/o

(Age x 3) + 7 = Weight (kg)

Fluid Resuscitation Guidelines: Burns:

Burn + Signs/Symptoms of Shock = 20 mL/kg

Parkland Formula: % Burn Surface Area x Weight (kg) ÷ 4 = mL/hr each hour x 8 hours

Drip Rate Formula:
1 IV/IO Site: %Burn Surface Area x Weight (kg) x 4 ÷ 100 = drops/minute (10 drop set)
2 IV/IO Sites: %Burn Surface Area x Weight (kg) x 2 ÷ 100 = drops/minute (10 drop set)

Pediatric Endotracheal Tube Guidelines:

Tube Size (mm) = (Age ÷ 4) + 4

Tube Depth (cm)

- < 1 y/o: Weight ÷ 2 + 8
- > 1 y/o: Age ÷ 2 + 13

Causes of Respiratory Deterioration (D.O.P.E.)

- Displacement
- Obstruction
- Pneumothorax
- Equipment

Pediatric Cardiac Arrest

```
┌─────────────────────────┐
│ Pulseless or Pulse <60  │
└─────────────────────────┘
            ↓
```

Initiate High Quality CPR
Push hard: > 1/3 diameter of chest
Push fast: 100-125 compressions
Allow full chest recoil
2 Rescuer 15:2
Advanced Airway: 1 breath every 6-8 sec.
Rotate compressors every 2 min.

↓

Attach cardiac monitor
Administer oxygen

Assess rhythm/glucose →

V-Fib/Pulseless V-Tach

- Shock 2 J/kg
- CPR 2 min.
- IV/IO
- Shock 4 J/kg
- CPR 2 min.
- Advanced Airway
- Epinephrine
- Shock 6 J/kg
- CPR 2 min.
- Amiodarone
- Shock 8 J/kg
- CPR 2 min.
- Epinephrine
- Shock 10 J/kg (max:360)
- CPR 2 min.
- Amiodarone
- Shock
- CPR 2 min.
- Epinephrine
- Shock
- CPR 2 min.
- Amiodarone
- Shock/CPR/Epinephrine

Asystole/PEA

- CPR 2 min.
- IV/IO
- Epinephrine
- Advanced Airway
- CPR
- Epinephrine

Dextrose 10: 1 mL/kg (0.5 G/kg) + 4 x volume in mL NS
Dextrose 25: 1 mL/kg (0.5 G/kg) + 1 x volume in mL NS

Epinephrine 1:10,000: 0.1 mL/kg (0.01 mg/kg) IV/IO
Epinephrine 1:1000: 0.1 mL/kg (0.1 mg/kg) ET+2 mL NS

Amiodarone: 0.1 mL/kg (5 mg/kg) IV/IO

Narcan: 0.1 mL/kg (0.1 mg/kg) IV/IO/ET

Sodium Bicarbonate: 1 mL/kg (1 mEQ/kg) + 1 mL/kg NS

Fluid Bolus: 20 mL/kg

Glucagon: 0.1 mL/kg
minimum: 0.5 mL

Atropine: 0.2 mL/kg (.02mg/kg)
minimum 0.1 mg (1 mL)
maximum 0.5 mg (5 mL)

Calcium: 2 mL/kg (20 mg/kg)

Causes of Cardiac Arrest

- Hypovolemia
- Hypoxia
- Hypothermia
- Hypoglycemia
- Hypokalemia
- Hyperkalemia
- Acidosis
- Tension Pneumo
- Tamponade
- Toxins
- Thrombosis

Pediatric Bradycardia

Cardiac monitor
Administer oxygen
Maintain airway
Assess glucose
IV/IO Access
12 Lead ECG

Treat underlying cause

Heart rate < 60/min

- Positive pressure ventilation
- CPR

Epinephrine 1:10,000: 0.1 mL/kg (0.01 mg/kg) IV/IO
Epinephrine 1:1000: 0.1 mL/kg (0.1 mg/kg) ET+2 mL NS

Fluid Bolus: 20 mL/kg

Medical Control Consultation:

- Atropine: 0.2 mL/kg (.02mg/kg)
  minimum 0.1 mg (1 mL) maximum 0.5 mg (5 mL)
- Transcutaneous Pacing

Pediatric Tachycardia

Cardiac monitor
Administer oxygen
Maintain airway
Assess glucose
IV/IO Access
12 Lead ECG

Treat underlying cause

Sinus Tachycardia

- QRS <0.08 sec
- Infant: < 220/min
- Child: < 180/min

PSVT

- QRS < 0.08 sec (2 boxes)
- Infant: > 220/min
- Child: > 180/min

Wide Complex Tachycardia

- QRS > 0.08 sec (2 boxes)
- Infant: >220/min
- Child: > 180/min

Fluid Bolus: 20 mL/kg

Stable

- Vagal Maneuver
  Apply ice pack to face
- Fluid Bolus: 20 mL/kg
- Adenosine

Stable and Monomorphic

- Fluid Bolus: 20 mL/kg
- Adenosine
- Amiodarone

Unstable:

- Versed
- Synchronized Cardioversion 1 J/kg
- Synchronized Cardioversion 2 J/kg

Adenosine

- 1st dose: 0.033 mL/kg (0.1 mg/kg)
- 2nd dose: 0.066 mL/kg (0.2 mg/kg)

Amiodarone

- 0.1 mL/kg (5 mg/kg) over 20 min
  Mix in 100 mL NS: 50 drops/min
  (10 drop set)

Versed

- 1:1 concentration: 0.2 mL/kg (0.2 mg/kg)
- 5:1 concentration: 0.04 mL/kg (0.2 mg/kg)

Neonatal Resuscitation

Warm and vigorously dry infant

Position infant to open airway:

(padding beneath shoulder blades)

Clamp and cut umbilical cord.

Suction airway if excessive secretions and signs of respiratory compromise are present.

Stimulate: massage infant's back or gently strike the soles of infant's feet.

Respirations:

- Inadequate or gasping: Positive pressure ventilations at 40-60 breaths/min./oxygen
- Shallow or slow: Administer oxygen for one minute. If respirations do not increase, provide positive pressure ventilations at 40-60 breaths/min./oxygen

Heart Rate:

- < 60: Chest compressions at 120/min.
- Compression to Ventilation Ratio 3:1

Advanced Airway (one attempt):

- Apnea
- Central cyanosis
- Bradycardia (<100)

IV/IO Access:

- Pulse < 60: IV/IO Epinephrine 1:10,000 0.01 mg/kg (0.3 mL; 0.03 mg)
  ET Epinephrine 1:1000 0.1 mg/kg (0.3 mL + 2.7 mL Normal Saline)
- Fluid Bolus: 30-60 mL Normal Saline
- Glucose < 60: Dextrose 10% 0.5 G/kg (3 mL D50W + 12 mL Normal Saline)

Adult Drug Calculations:

Adenosine: 1st dose: 6 mg (2 mL)   2nd dose: 12 mg (4 mL)   concentration: 6 mg/2 mL

Amiodarone:
V-Fib/Pulseless V-Tach: 1st dose: 300 mg (6 mL) 2nd dose: 150 mg (3 mL); concentration: 150 mg/ 3mL

Amiodarone: V-Tach with Pulse: 150 mg (3 mL) over 10 min. ; Maintenance Drip: 1 mg /min
[100 mg (2 mL)/100 mL NS]

Atropine: 0.5 mg (5 mL) Cumulative dose: 3 mg concentration: 1 mg/10 mL

Benadryl: 50 mg (1 mL) concentration: 50 mg/mL

Calcium Chloride: 1000 mg (10 mL) Slow IVP concentration: 1000 mg/10 mL

Dextrose 50%: 25 G (50 mL) concentration 25 G/50 mL (0.5 G/mL)

Dopamine: 5-10 mcg/kg/min concentration 1600 mcg/mL

Epinephrine: 1 mg concentration: 1 mg/10 mL

Epinephrine 1:1000: ET: 2 mg concentration: 1 mg/mL

Epinephrine 1:1000: SQ/IM: 0.3 mg (0.3 mL) concentration: 1 mg/mL   Epi-Pen (0.3 mg)

Epinephrine: Nebulized: 5 mL Epi 1:1000 (5 mg)

Fentanyl: 50 (1 mL)-200 (4 mL) mcg   concentration: 50 mcg/mL

Glucagon: 1 mg (1 mL)   concentration: 1 mg/mL

Haldol: 5 mg (1 mL) IM Only concentration: 5 mg/mL

Lidocaine: 1 mg/kg (0.05 mL/kg) concentration: 100 mg/5 mL

Magnesium Sulfate:
concentration: 1 G/2 mL: Mix 4 mL (2000 mg) Mag Sulfate + 100 mL NS: 100 drops/min.; 10 drop set
concentration: 2 G/50 mL: 50 drops/min.; 10 drop set

Morphine: Mix 5 mg/mL Morphine in 9 mL NS: 2.5 mg (5 mL)-5 mg (10 mL)   concentration: 1 mg/2mL

Narcan: 2 mg (2 mL)   concentration 2 mg/2 mL

Sodium Bicarbonate: 1 mEq/kg (1 mL/kg)   concentration 1 mEq/mL

Solumedrol: 125 mg   concentration 62.5 mg/mL

Adult Drug Calculations

Valium: IV/IO/IO: 2 mg (0.4 mL) -10 mg (2 mL)   concentration: 5 mg/mL

Versed:
concentration: 1 mg/mL: 2.5 mg (2.5 mL)- 5 mg (5 mL)
concentration: 5 mg/mL: 2.5 mg (0.5 mL)-5 mg (1 mL)

Zofran: Mix 2 mL (4 mg) Zofran + 2 mL NS: Slow IVP   concentration: 2 mg/mL

BVM: Tidal volume: 7 mL/kg   ETT: 7.0 – 9.0   Depth: 21-24 cm   Supraglottic Airway: #3, #4, #5

OPA: 80 mm, 90 mm, 100 mm, 110 mm   NPA: 30-36 F

Dopamine [60 drop set]

5 mcg/kg/min:

50 kg	9 drops/min
75 kg	14 drops/min
100 kg	19 drops/min
125 kg	23 drops/min
150 kg	28 drops/min
175 kg	33 drops/min
200 kg	38 drops/min
225 kg	42 drops/min
250 kg	47 drops/min
300 kg	56 drops/min

10 mcg/kg/min

50 kg	19 drops/min
75 kg	28 drops/min
100 kg	38 drops/min
125 kg	47 drops/min
150 kg	56 drops/min
175 kg	66 drops/min
200 kg	75 drops/min
225 kg	84 drops/min
250 kg	94 drops/min
300 kg	113 drops/min

15 mcg/kg/min

50 kg	28 drops/min
75 kg	42 drops/min
100 kg	56 drops/min
125 kg	70 drops/min
150 kg	84 drops/min
175 kg	98 drops/min
200 kg	113 drops/min
225 kg	127 drops/min
250 kg	141 drops/min
300 kg	169 drops/min

Epinephrine

*Cardiogenic Hypotension:

2-10 mcg/min.

Mix 1 mL (1 mg) Epi 1:1000 in 100 mL NS

Concentration: 1000 mcg/100 mL 10 :1

(10 mcg/mL)

[60 drop set]

2.5 mcg/min= 15 drops

5 mcg/min= 30 drops

7.5 mcg/min= 45 drops

10 mcg/min= 60 drops

Mix 4 mL (4 mg) Epi 1:1000 in 1000 mL NS

Concentration: 4000 mcg/1000 mL 4:1

(4 mcg/mL)

[60 drop set]

2 mcg/min= 30 drops

4 mcg/min= 60 drops

6 mcg/min= 90 drops

8 mcg/min= 120 drops

10 mcg/min= 150 drops

*Anaphylaxis [10 drop set]

5 mL/min (50 mcg/min) = 50 drops/min

Magnesium Sulfate

*Pre-eclampsia/Asthma/COPD

2 Grams/50 mL over 10 minutes

- 10 drop set: 50 drops/min
- 60 drop set: 300 drops/min

or

Mix 2 Grams (4 mL) in 100 mL NS

- 10 drop set: 100 drops/min
- 60 drop set: 600 drops/min

*Post Conversion: Polymorphic V-Tach: 1-4 mg/min

Mix 4 Grams (8 mL) in 1000 mL NS [60 drop set]

- 1 mg/min: 15 drops/min
- 2 mg/min: 30 drops/min
- 3 mg/min: 45 drops/min
- 4 mg/min: 60 drops/min

Amiodarone

150 mg over 10 minutes

Mix 3 mL (150 mg) in 100 mL NS

- 10 drop set: 100 drops/min
- 60 drop set: 600 drops/min

Maintenance Drip: 1 mg/min.

Mix 2 mL (100 mg) in 100 mL NS

- 10 drop set: 10 drops/min
- 60 drop set: 60 drops/min

Lidocaine

1-4 mg/min [60 drop set]

- 1 mg/min: 15 drops/min
- 2 mg/min: 30 drops/min
- 3 mg/min: 45 drops/min
- 4 mg/min: 60 drops/min

Left Hemisphere Stroke Syndrome

- Right Side Weakness/Right Arm Drift
- Right Facial Droop
- Right Sensory Deficit
- Right Visual Deficit
- Aphasia: inability to speak, incorrect phrase or word patterns, inability to comprehend language
- Eyes Gaze Left

Right Hemisphere Stroke Syndrome

- Left Side Weakness/Left Arm Drift
- Left Facial Droop
- Left Sensory Deficit
- Left Visual Deficit
- Left Side Neglect: unaware of left side
- Eyes Gaze Right

Brainstem Stroke Syndrome

- Decreased Level of Consciousness
- Nausea/Vomiting
- Abnormal Respiratory Pattern
- Double Vision
- Dysconjugate Gaze: failure of the eyes to move in the same direction
- Nystagmus: jerking eye movements
- Dysphagia: difficulty swallowing
- Dysarthria: difficulty speaking: slurred or slow speech pattern
- Sensory Deficits on Both Sides of Body
- Bilateral Facial Droop
- Bilateral Arm Drift
- Contralateral Weakness: one side of face is weak; opposite side of body is weak

Cerebellum Stroke Syndrome

- Abnormal Gait: Gait Ataxia: unbalanced while standing with wide gait
- Dysequilibrium
- Dyscoordination: "finger to nose/heel to shin test abnormal

Subarachnoid Hemorrhagic Stroke

- Headache
- Nausea/Vomiting
- Decreased Level of Consciousness
- Intolerance to Light
- Neck Pain/Stiffness

Intracerebral Hemorrhagic Stroke

- Headache
- Nausea/Vomiting
- Decreased Level of Consciousness
- Hemiparesis: weakness on one side of the body

Myocardial Infarction: 12/15 Lead

Inferior Infarct:

- ST Elevation: II, III, aVF
- ST Depression: I, aVL,   V5, V6
- Perform Right-side ECG (Move V4 to opposite side of chest)
- ST Elevation in V4R= Right Ventricular Involvement

- *Oxygen
  *Aspirin
  * Normal Saline Fluid Bolus 250 mL (may be repeated)
  *Dopamine 2-10 mcg/kg/min; Epi Drip 2-10 mcg/min. (Hypotension refractory to fluid bolus)
  *No NTG
  *No Morphine

Inferior-Posterior Infarct: High Index of Suspicion for Dissecting Aortic Aneurysm:

- ST Elevation: II, III, aVF
- ST Depression: I, aVL,   V1, V2,   V3, V4,   V5, V6
- Right-side ECG: ST Elevation: V4R
- 15 Lead ECG: ST Elevation: V8, V9
- History of Hypertension : 99% probability of aneurysm
  *IV/IO Access
  *Oxygen

  *No NTG
  *No Fluid Bolus
  *No Morphine

Lateral Infarct:

- ST Elevation: I, aVL, V5, V6
- ST Depression: II, III, aVF
  *Oxygen
  *Aspirin
- BP >110
  *NTG
  *Morphine

NTG Contraindications:

- Use of Erectile Dysfunction Medications
- BP < 110
- Tachycardia
- Bradycardia
- Inferior Infarct with Right Ventricle Involved

Myocardial Infarction: 12/15 Lead ECG

Inferior-Posterior Infarct:

- ST Elevation: II, III, aVF
- ST Depression: I, aVL, V5, V6
- ST Depression: V1, V2 V3, V4
- Right-side ECG: No ST Elevation in V4R
- 15 Lead ECG: ST Elevation V8, V9
- No Previous History of Hypertension
  *Oxygen
  *Aspirin
  *Normal Saline Fluid Bolus 250 mL (may be repeated)
- BP >110
  * NTG (Consult Medical Control)
  * Morphine (Consult Medical Control)

Posterior Infarct:

- ST Depression: V1, V2 V3, V4
- 15 Lead ECG: ST Elevation: V8, V9
  *Oxygen
  *Aspirin
- BP >110
  *NTG
  *Morphine

Anterior Infarct:

- ST Elevation: V3, V4
  *Oxygen
  *Aspirin
- BP >110
  *NTG
  *Morphine

Septal Infarct:

- ST Elevation: V1, V2
  *Oxygen
  *Aspirin
- BP >110
  *NTG
  *Morphine

NTG Contraindications:

- Use of Erectile Dysfunction Medications
- BP < 110
- Tachycardia
- Bradycardia
- Inferior Infarct with Right Ventricle Involved

Causes of Cardiac Arrest: * Signs and Corrective Actions

- Hypovolemia: Fluid Bolus

- Hypoxia: Airway/Oxygen/Ventilation

- Hydrogen Ion Acidosis: Sodium Bicarbonate

- Hypokalemia
  *Flat T-Waves, U-Waves, Wide QRS

- Hyperkalemia: Calcium Chloride, Sodium Bicarbonate, Nebulized Albuterol
  *Tall, Peaked T-Waves, Wide QRS

- Hypoglycemia: Dextrose

- Hypothermia: Warming

- Toxins: Narcan (Opiates), Sodium Bicarbonate(Tricyclics)
  Glucagon/Calcium Chloride (Beta-Blockers, Calcium Channel Blockers)

- Tamponade
  *Tachycardia, Narrow QRS, JVD

- Tension Pneumothorax: Chest Decompression
  *Bradycardia, Narrow QRS, JVD, Tracheal Deviation, Unilateral Breath Sounds, Poor
  BVM Compliance, No Pulse Felt With CPR

- Thrombosis: MI
  *ST Elevation in 2 Contiguous Leads

- Thrombosis: PE
  *Tachycardia, Narrow QRS, JVD, No Pulse Felt With CPR

Revised Trauma Score

	Glasgow Coma Scale	Systolic B/P	Respirations
4	13-15	>89	10-29
3	9-12	76-89	>29
2	6-8	50-75	6-9
1	4-5	<50	1-5
0	3	0	0

Pediatric Trauma Score

	+ 2	+ 1	-1
Weight (kg)	>20	10-20	<10
Airway	Patent	Maintainable	Non-Maintainable
Systolic BP	>90	50-90	<50
Mental Status	Awake	Altered	Unresponsive
Open Wound/Bleeding	None	Minor	Major
Extremity Fracture	None	Closed/Singular	Open or Multiple

Spinal Motion Restriction

National Emergency X-Ray Utilization Study (NEXUS) Criteria:

- No posterior midline cervical spine tenderness.

- No evidence of intoxication.

- No altered mental status.

- No focal neurological deficit.

- No painful distracting injuries.

Fluid Resuscitation Guideline: Burns

- Burn + Signs of Shock = Fluid Bolus
- EMS Parkland Formula: Burn Surface Area % x Weight (kg) x 0.25 = mL/hr for the first 8 hours
- EMS Burn Infusion: Burn Surface Area % x Weight (kg) x 0.04 = drops/minute ÷ # of IV/IO Sites

Trauma Triage Criteria

Physiologic:

Glasgow Coma Scale	< 13
Systolic Blood Pressure	< 90
Respiratory Rate	Adult: <10 or >29; Infant < 20/ Need for positive pressure ventilations.

Anatomic:

Penetrating injury to head, neck, torso, extremities proximal to elbow or knee
Chest wall instability or deformity (flail chest)
Two or more proximal long bone fractures
Crushed, degloved, mangles, or pulseless extremity
Amputation proximal to wrist or ankle
Pelvic fractures
Open or depressed skull fracture
Paralysis

Mechanism:

Falls • Adults: > 20 feet • Pediatric: >10 feet or 2-3 times the height of the child.
High-Risk Auto Collision • Intrusion >12 inches in occupant site or 18 inches any site • Ejection (partial or complete) • Death in same passenger compartment • Vehicle telemetry data consistent with high risk of injury
Auto vs. Pedestrian/Bicyclist • Thrown, run-over, significant impact • > 20 mph
Motorcycle Crash • > 20 mph

Special Considerations:

Older Adults • Risk of injury/death increases > 65 years of age. • Systolic BP <110 may represent shock > 65 years of age. • Low impact mechanisms (ground level fall) may result in severe injury.
Pregnancy • > 20 weeks
Anticoagulants and Bleeding Disorders • Patients with head injury are at high risk for rapid deterioration.
EMS Provider Judgment

Triage

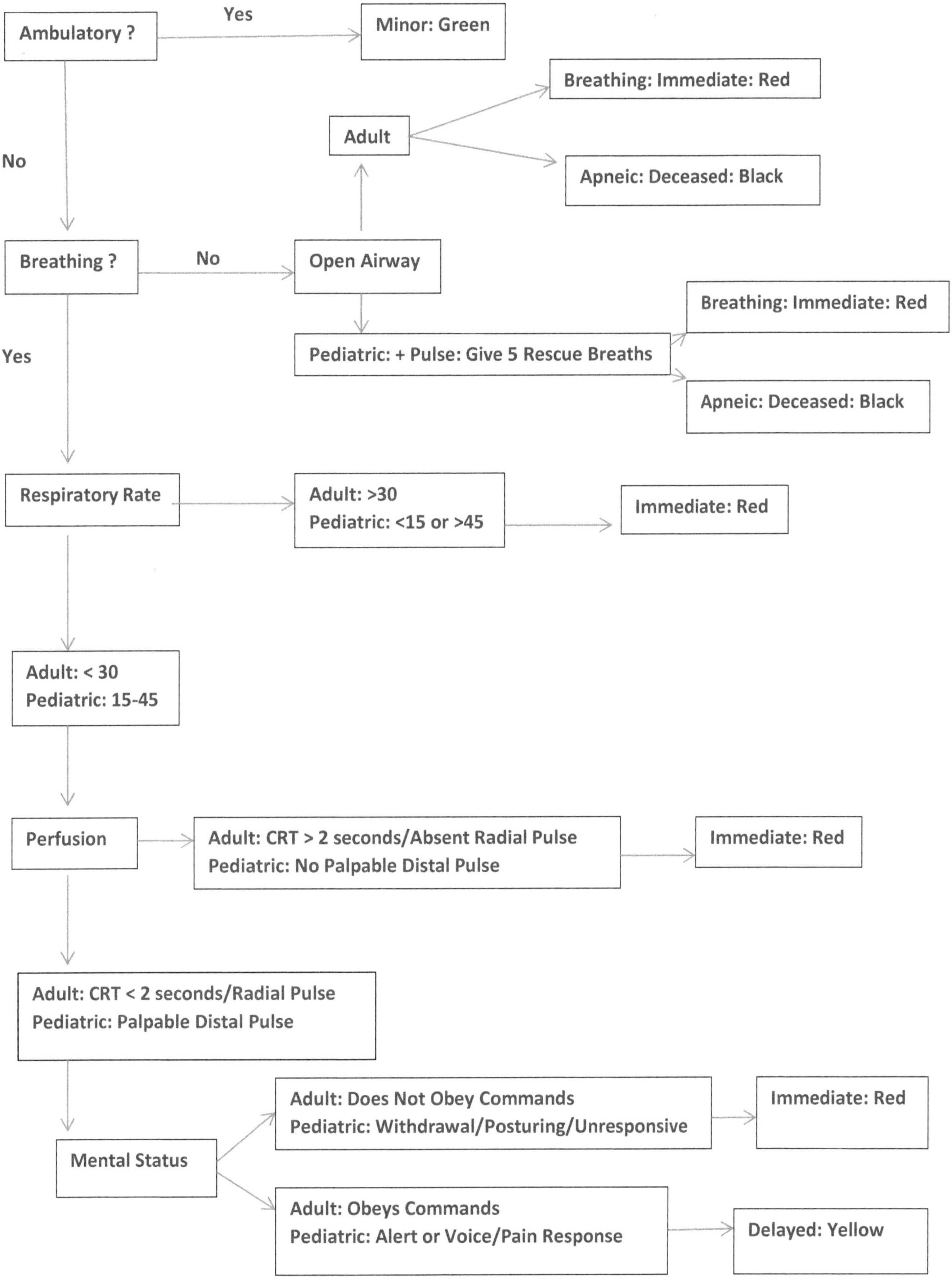

```
Ambulatory ? ──── Yes ────▶ Minor: Green
     │
     │ No
     │
     ▼
```

```
                                          ┌─▶ Breathing: Immediate: Red
                              Adult ───────┤
                                          └─▶ Apneic: Deceased: Black
```

```
Breathing ? ──── No ────▶ Open Airway ────▶ Adult
     │                          │
     │ Yes                      ▼
     │              Pediatric: + Pulse: Give 5 Rescue Breaths
     │                                          ├─▶ Breathing: Immediate: Red
     │                                          └─▶ Apneic: Deceased: Black
     ▼
```

```
Respiratory Rate ────▶ Adult: >30          ────▶ Immediate: Red
     │                 Pediatric: <15 or >45
     ▼
```

```
Adult: < 30
Pediatric: 15-45
     │
     ▼
```

```
Perfusion ────▶ Adult: CRT > 2 seconds/Absent Radial Pulse ────▶ Immediate: Red
     │          Pediatric: No Palpable Distal Pulse
     ▼
```

```
Adult: CRT < 2 seconds/Radial Pulse
Pediatric: Palpable Distal Pulse
     │
     ▼
```

```
Mental Status ───┬─▶ Adult: Does Not Obey Commands              ────▶ Immediate: Red
                 │   Pediatric: Withdrawal/Posturing/Unresponsive
                 │
                 └─▶ Adult: Obeys Commands                       ────▶ Delayed: Yellow
                     Pediatric: Alert or Voice/Pain Response
```

Post Resuscitation:

- Oxygenation: titrate to maintain 94%
- Capnometry: adjust ventilations to maintain 35-45 mm/Hg

- Was the patient ever in V-Fib or Pulseless V-Tach?
  Yes: Amiodarone 150 mg (3 mL) in 100 mL NS over 10 minutes.(100 drops/min: 10 drop set)

- Was the patient in Torsades de Pointes?
- Yes: Magnesium Sulfate 1-4 mg/min. (4 Grams in 1000 mL NS)(15-60 drops/min: 60 drop set)

- Is the patient responsive?
  No: Therapeutic Hypothermia:
  *cold packs placed in axillae and groin

  Contraindications:
  * suspected intracranial hemorrhage
  * severe hemorrhage
  * hypotension refractory to multiple vasopressors
  * sepsis
  * pregnancy
  * pulmonary edema

- Perform 12 Lead ECG
  STEMI: Transport to PCI Facility

- Support Blood Pressure
  *Dopamine 5-10 mcg/kg/min [(5-10 x kg x 6) ÷ 160] = drops/min.

  *Epinephrine 0.1-0.5 mcg/kg/min (1 mg in 100 mL NS) [0.1 x kg x 6 = drops/min] (60 drop set)
  [0.25-0.5 x kg = drops/min] (10 drop set)

Devotional For Emergency Responders

Firefighting

"We might be thrown into the blazing furnace, but the God we serve is able to bring us out of it alive." *-Daniel 3:17*

"They came out of the fire and the fire had not harmed them." *-Daniel 3:26-27*

"You will walk through fire, but you will not be burned." *-Isaiah 43:2*

"The fire will test how good everyone's work is. If the building doesn't burn up, God will provide reward. If the building burns up, the builder will lose everything, but God will save."
-1 Corinthians 3:13-15

"Suppose I give my body to be burned. If I don't have love, I get nothing at all."
-1 Corinthians 13:3

"They put out great fires. Their weakness was turned to strength." *-Hebrews 11:34*

"Pull others out of the fire. Save them." *-Jude 1:23*

"Fire tests silver. Heat tests gold. But the LORD tests the heart." *-Proverbs 27:1*

Patient Care

"They will place their hands on sick people and the people will get well." *-Mark 16:18*

"Then He sent them out to preach about God's Kingdom and to heal those who were sick."
-Luke 9:2

" When you enter a town, heal the sick people who are there." *-Luke 10:8-9*

"When he saw the man, he bandaged his wounds." *-Luke 10:33*

"God has appointed people who have the gift of healing and are able to help others."
-1 Corinthians 12:28

Courage

"Be strong and courageous. The Lord your God will go with you. He will never leave you. He will never desert you." -Deuteronomy 31:6

"Be strong and brave. Do not be terrified. Do not lose hope. I Am the Lord your God. I will be with you everywhere you go." -Joshua 1:9

"Even though I walk through the valley of the shadow of death, I will have no fear. God is with me." -Psalm 23:4

"The Lord gives me light and saves me. Why should I fear anyone? The Lord is my place of safety. Why should I be afraid?"   -Psalm 27:1

"God didn't give us a spirit that makes us weak and fearful. He gave us a spirit that gives us power and love."   -2 Timothy 1:7

Service

"Also work for the success of the city I have sent you to. Pray to the Lord for that city. If it succeeds, you too will enjoy success." -Jeremiah 29:7

"In the same way, let your light shine in front of others. Then they will see the good things you do and they will praise your Father, Who is in heaven." -Matthew 5:16

"We know that in all things God works for the good of those who love Him and are called according to His purpose." -Romans 8:28

"Carry each other's heavy loads." -Galatians 6:2

"Work at everything you do with all your heart. Work as if you were working for the Lord." -Colossians 3:23

" Don't just talk about love. Put your love into action." - 1 John 3:18

" Suppose someone forces you to go one mile. Go two miles with him." -Matthew 5:41

Friendship

" Jesus said, 'For where two or three come together in My Name, there am I with them.'"
-Matthew 18:20

" As iron sharpens iron, so one man sharpens another." -Proverbs 27:17

" Two are better than one, because they have a good return for their work:
If one falls down, his friend can help him up." - Ecclesiastes 4:9-10

" Therefore encourage one another and build each other up, just as in fact you are doing."
-1 Thessalonians 5:11

" Show proper respect for everyone; love the brotherhood; fear God; honor the king."
-1 Peter 2:17

" Finally, all of you, live in harmony with one another; be sympathetic, love one another like members of the same family, be compassionate and humble." - 1 Peter 3:8

" Love each other deeply. Honor others more than yourself. Never let the fire in your heart go out. Keep it alive. Serve the Lord."   -Romans 12:10-11

Tragedy

"The Lord is close to those whose hearts have been broken. He saves those whose spirits have been crushed."   -Psalm 34:18

"Trust in the Lord with all your heart and lean not on your own understanding"   -Proverbs 3:5

"The Lord's ways are higher than our ways. The Lord's thoughts are higher than our thoughts." -Isaiah 55:9

"In this world you will have trouble. But take heart! Jesus has overcome the world."
-John 16:33

"I'm glad when I am weak. I'm glad in hard times. I'm glad when people say mean things about me. I'm glad when things are difficult. I'm glad when people make me suffer. When I am weak, I am strong."   -2 Corinthians 12:10

"My brothers and sisters, you will face all kinds of trouble. When you do, think of it as pure joy. Your faith will be put to the test. You know when that happens it will produce in you the strength to endure." -James 1:2-4

"Jesus will wipe away every tear. There will be no more death or sadness. There will be no more crying or pain. Things will no longer be the way they used to be."   -Revelation 21:4

Salvation

" He was pierced for our transgressions, He was crushed for our iniquities, the punishment that brought us peace was upon Him, and by His wounds we are healed." -Isaiah 53:5

" For God so loved the world that He gave His only begotten Son, that whoever believes in Him shall not perish, but have eternal life." -John 3:16

" Jesus said, 'I am the way, the truth, and the life. No one comes to the Father except through Me.'" -John 14:6

" For all have sinned and fall short of the glory of God." - Romans 3:23

" God demonstrates His own love for us in this: While we were still sinners, Christ died for us." -Romans 5:8

" For the wages of sin is death, but the gift of God is eternal life in Jesus Christ our Lord." -Romans 6:23

" That if you confess with your mouth, 'Jesus is Lord,' and believe in your heart that God raised Him from the dead, you will be saved." -Romans 10-9